# NURSING THE PERSON WITH CANCER

## A book for all nurses

*Edited by* Gordon Poulton

*Foreword by* Laurie Grealish

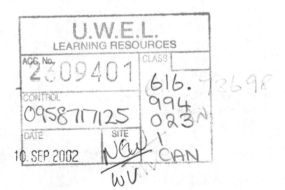
AUSMED PUBLICATIONS
MELBOURNE

*Australasian Health Education Systems Pty Ltd*
*(ACN 005 611 626)*
*trading as*
*Ausmed Publications*
*275–277 Mount Alexander Road*
*Ascot Vale, Victoria 3032, Australia*

First published March 1998

Further copies of this book and of all other Ausmed publications are available from the Distribution Manager, Ausmed Publications, PO Box 4086, Melbourne University, Victoria 3052, Australia.
Telephone +61 3 9375 7311.
Fax +61 3 9375 7299.
E-mail ausmed@ausmed.com.au
Home page www.ausmed.com.au

National Library of Australia Cataloguing-in-Publication data:
Nursing the person with cancer : a book for all nurses

Includes index
ISBN 0 9587171 2 5.

1.     Cancer – Nursing. I Poulton, Gordon, 1955- .

610.73698

Edited by Robyn Whiteley and John Collins, The WC Company Pty Ltd

Cover, design and typesetting by Colorperception Pty Ltd

Text set in 10/12 Garamond

Printed in Australia by Hyde Park Press

# Foreword

*Laurie Grealish*

Two in every three Australians will be touched by cancer in their lifetimes, either personally or through a close family member. Cancer has a historical reputation for being a killer disease, a death sentence. This is reflected in the colloquial meanings attributed to the word 'cancer'. Although most types of cancer have eluded a medical cure, more than 50 per cent of people diagnosed with cancer today go on to live for five years or more. This has meant a partial shift in nursing practice, to including rehabilitation along with acute care and palliation as a care delivery model. Cancer is a chronic illness managed by multidisciplinary teams in the same way as diabetes and arthritis. Although it has continued to hold its terrifying power, a cancer diagnosis can be managed by patients and their families with the support of the nurse.

On first glance, the chapters of this book appear to have no clear connection. There is no reference to the systems of the body, the stages of disease, the types of medical treatment, or the technical care of the person with cancer. Rather, each chapter discloses information that cannot be readily found in standard cancer nursing textbooks. This books reflects the widely held view that cancer nursing is more than medically related care. It focuses on the person, what the experience of cancer means to that person, and how the nurse can help. Communication is the continuous thread that links each chapter.

The communication skills of the nurse are invaluable in guiding individuals and families along their journey through the cancer experience. The communication skills required in caring for those experiencing cancer are not specialist skills; they are the simple skills of listening, reflecting, and providing accurate information. All registered nurses possess these skills.

By reading the chapters in this book, the nurse will be exposed to refreshing perspectives on the cancer experience. The ideas raised in the book can be reflected on and discussed with colleagues for further development. The practical suggestions from many authors can be integrated into the practice of specialist and generalist alike, to improve the quality of nursing care for the person with cancer.

Cancer nursing is a fully fledged specialty in Australia as evidenced by the steady development of a unified national cancer nursing association, known as the Cancer Nurses Society of Australia. The appearance of this book is a sign that cancer nurses are confident to document and share their specialist experiences and knowledge. The authors in this book challenge each of us to expand our knowledge of the cancer experience and, through the application of basic communication skills, support persons and families throughout the cancer experience.

*Laurie Grealish*

Laurie Grealish
Registered Nurse, Master of Nursing, Oncology Certificate,
Fellow of the College of Nursing (New South Wales),
Fellow of the Royal College of Nursing, Australia
Lecturer in Nursing, University of Canberra
Chair, Clinical Oncological Society of Australia Nurses Group
Chair, Cancer Nurses Society of Australia Steering Committee
Member of Board, International Society of Nurses in Cancer Care

# Contents

Foreword — v

The cover — x

Dedication — xi

Acknowledgments — xii

**Section One**    Awareness or innocence: Explanation and education

*Chapter 1*    Dispelling myths, imparting knowledge — a guide to client education — 3
*Gordon Poulton*

*Chapter 2*    Challenges and opportunities — educating the nurse for cancer care — 13
*Sanchia Aranda*

*Chapter 3*    The importance of communication and the provision of information in patient care — 27
*Doreen Akkerman*

*Chapter 4*    Breaking bad news — 39
*Gordon Poulton*

**Section Two**    Tears and fears: The impact of diagnosis

*Chapter 5*    Hope — the inner strength — 51
*Judy Zollo*

*Chapter 6*    Cancer and sexuality — a neglected issue? — 64
*Stephanie Wellard* and *Trish Joyce*

*Chapter 7*    Cancer pain — providing solutions for current problems — 88
*Lera O'Connor*

**Section Three**    The challenge: Issues for nurses

*Chapter 8*    Assessing and knowing the person with cancer — 109
*Beverleigh Quested*

| | | |
|---|---|---|
| **Chapter 9** | Caring<br>*Louise Nicholson* | 123 |
| **Chapter 10** | Ethical challenges for cancer nurses<br>*Julie Cairns* | 137 |
| **Chapter 11** | Spirituality — the essence of cancer care<br>*Tony Bush* | 149 |
| **Chapter 12** | Palliative care — an integrated part of<br>cancer care<br>*Alison McLeod* and *Karen Glaetzer* | 163 |
| **Chapter 13** | Caregiver support<br>*Cameron Sinclair* | 175 |
| **Chapter 14** | Multiculturalism — implications for<br>cancer care<br>*Lera O'Connor* | 187 |
| **Chapter 15** | Exploring the boundries of oncological<br>nursing practice<br>*Marie Cuddihy* | 199 |
| **Section Four** | Examples of Australian research | |
| Research piece A | Lymphoedema<br>*Jennifer Green* | 210 |
| Research piece B | Breast cancer diagnosis —<br>detection methods<br>and emotions experienced<br>*Linda Reaby* | 218 |
| Research piece C | Adcare Lifestyle Retreat —<br>empowerment and enrichment<br>for people living with cancer<br>*Anne Fowler, Gloria Swift* and<br>*Lucia Apolloni* | 228 |
| Research piece D | What CanTeen patients think about their<br>treatment<br>*Anthony Cammell* | 235 |
| **Index** | | 241 |

# Illustrations

Figures
| | | |
|---|---|---|
| 4.1 | Breaking bad news | 41 |
| 4.2 | Handling the effects of bad news | 42 |
| 6.1 | The hypothalamic, pituitary, gonadal axis | 68 |
| 7.1 | The concept of suffering | 91 |
| 7.2 | The WHO 3-step analgesic ladder for cancer pain | 94 |
| 7.3 | Analgesic ladder for cancer pain management based on diagnosis of origin of the pain | 95 |
| 7.4 | Pain intensity rating scales | 97 |
| 8.1 | Summary of elements in knowing patients | 111 |
| C.1 | Questions asked of Adcare participants involved in the 1997 retreat | 231 |

Tables
| | | |
|---|---|---|
| 2.1 | Curriculum and self-study guide for core concepts in cancer nursing | 16 |
| 2.2 | Opportunities in the 21st century | 21 |
| 6.1 | Chemotherapeutic agents affecting sexual or reproductive function | 70 |
| 6.2 | Annon model of approaches to sexual concerns | 82 |
| 7.1 | Facts and fallacies about pain control | 93 |
| 7.2 | A patient diary | 99 |
| 7.3 | Non-pharmacologic methods of pain control | 101 |
| 7.4 | Analgesics used in cancer pain management | 103 |
| 7.5 | Side effects of morphine | 104 |
| 10.1 | SPIRAL model for decision-making | 142 |
| 15.1 | Characteristics of the emerging health care system in the USA | 201 |
| 15.2 | Tenets of an assertive philosophy | 204 |
| A.1 | Perceived sequelae of lymphoedema | 213 |
| B.1 | Initial methods of breast cancer detection | 220 |
| B.2 | Feelings when diagnosed with breast cancer | 222 |
| B.3 | Fears when diagnosed with breast cancer | 223 |

# The cover

The cover of this book is taken from an original piece of artwork by Pierrette Nicole Boustany entitled 'In Memory of Yaya'. The work first appeared in an exhibition, *Cancer: The Journey,* held in the VicHealth Access Gallery of the National Gallery of Victoria, in Melbourne, Australia, 9–31 August 1996. Sponsored by the Anti-Cancer Council of Victoria, the exhibition featured works of art reflecting people's experience with cancer. The image is used with permission of the artist.

Pierrette's image was accompanied by the following words:

### IN MEMORY OF YAYA, MY GRANDMOTHER
### AN AMAZON OF THE 20TH CENTURY

*One day the unthinkable happened. Yaya was called upon to become an initiate of the 20th century Amazon tribe. Like all initiations, the coming times were filled with fear, pain and uncertainty; all that was, was no longer.*

*Like the ancient Amazons the first ritual in this lengthy process was the removal of her breast so that her chances in the coming battles would be increased.*

*Yaya's only weapons were her inner strength and the will to survive. For many years she battled and survived her enemy.*

*Until one day her initiation was completed. She had now become a 20th century Amazon. Nothing could stop her.*

*Then the Amazons of the sky came to claim her. She was theirs now.*

*I often think of her; remembering the things she taught me, her caring nature, her strength against all odds.*

by Pierrette Nicole Boustany

Pierrette can be contacted at PO Box 247, Fairfield, Victoria 3078, Australia. Mobile telephone no. 0418 106 893

# Dedication

There are many people involved in the making of a book and each of them has a special interest in and feel for the book as it grows and develops. Two of the people involved in the production of this book felt that they would like to dedicate their work on the book to people who have inspired them.

Gordon Poulton, the Editor of the book, wrote the following dedication:

*I would like to dedicate this book to the people, their families and loved ones who are living with the disease called cancer; also to the nurses who, over many years, have moulded a speciality of nursing practice that focuses on client needs; and finally to all those who have taken the time to care.*

Cynthea Wellings, Publisher of the book and Director of Ausmed Publications, wishes to dedicate her involvement in the book to a nurse who was inspirational:

*I dedicate this book to Norma Bryan, a truly remarkable nurse and a former Director of Nursing of Royal District Nursing Service, Melbourne.*

# ACKNOWLEDGMENTS

No undertaking of this nature is done alone. There have been many people who have contributed directly and others who have contributed indirectly to the success of this project. I would like to acknowledge and extend my warmest thanks to the following people for their help and support:

- Cynthea Wellings, for giving me the chance to do this project;

- The writers of the chapters, whose willingness to share their research and expertise and give their cooperation made it a privilege to have them as colleagues;

- Robyn Whiteley and John Collins for their expertise, patience and guidance during the past months and for their hospitality, impromptu meals and photographic prowess;

- Stacey McEvoy for her ideas and support;

- Denise Spencer who, when I asked her to be scathing when reviewing my chapters, did exactly as I asked, and who has put up with me and supported me all the way;

- All my colleagues at the Peter MacCallum Cancer Institute who have lived with my moods while this project was being completed;

- Barry Hearn whose poignant comments made me see things in a different light; and, finally,

- My family, both in Ballarat and in Melbourne for their understanding and support throughout what is inevitably an all-consuming but exciting experience.

*Gordon Poulton*
January 1998

# SECTION ONE

## *Awareness or innocence:*
## *Explanation and education*

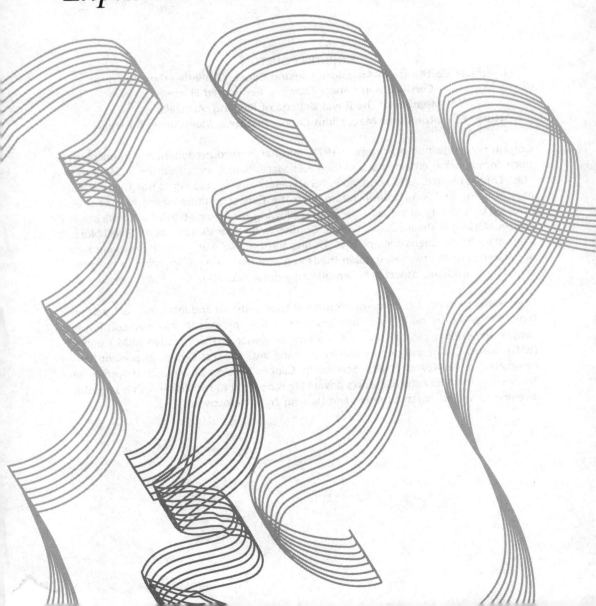

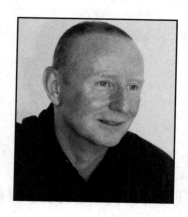

**GORDON POULTON**
**Graduate Certificate in Advanced Nursing Cancer/Palliative Care Nursing,**
**Certificate in Cancer Nursing, Registered Nurse,**
**Member of the Royal College of Nursing, Australia**
**Nurse Educator, Peter MacCallum Cancer Institute, Melbourne, Australia**

Gordon began his nursing career in 1979, and has worked predominantly in oncology since commencing employment at the Peter MacCallum Cancer Institute in 1980 as a State Enrolled Nurse. After completing his General Nursing Training at Box Hill Hospital in Melbourne in 1985, Gordon returned to the Cancer Institute where he has been involved in a variety of cancer care areas. Following the completion of a Certificate in Cancer Nursing at the Institute in 1988, Gordon worked for six years as a Clinical Nurse Consultant in the chemotherapy unit. During this time he was given the responsibility of coordinating the pilot Hospital in the Home program, and participating in both the clinical and academic aspects of chemotherapy nurse education.

Gordon has presented at numerous forums at local, national and international levels on topics ranging from nutrition in immunocompromised persons to informed consent in people undergoing clinical trials. He is a past convenor of the Victorian AIDS Council (VAC) Nurses Group and deputy convenor of the VAC Support Group. At present he is completing a Master of Health Science in Cancer Nursing at Victoria University of Technology in Melbourne. Gordon's private life is devoted to socialising with his friends, listening to a wide variety of music and tackling cryptic crosswords.

# Chapter 1

## Dispelling myths, imparting knowledge — a guide to client education

The art of educating people during their illness and recovery/rehabilitation period is an area in nursing that can be developed and improved as a nurse gains experience and maturity. Traditional nursing curricula have not always taught nurses *how* to educate. Certainly, when answering a question on an examination paper, a nurse could always gain an extra half mark by adding 'educate the patient' as a final point, but in reality education was not high on the list of identified nursing functions. This trend, however, is changing, and today most nursing faculties incorporate in their curricula subjects relating to client education, though they are not often given the priority they deserve with the result that they suffer from an 'education on the run' approach. Nolan (1995) points out ways that client education does not always follow established educational principles, for example, not allowing sufficient time for evaluation of the clients' level of understanding, knowledge and skills. Nolan claims this is particularly relevant in the education of people about their drug therapy. Often this is done on the day of discharge and Nolan points out that when the client is preoccupied with discharge procedures there is little hope of their even taking in information let alone having learning reinforced.

In recent times, many governments have focused on an illness prevention policy (Swerissen and Duckett, 1997). This is reflected in a statement published by the Public Health Association of Australia (Victorian Branch) which states that

> . . . the programmes, services, and institutions involved emphasize the prevention of disease and the health needs of the population as a whole.

In supporting a policy such as this, nurses have an opportunity to be at the forefront in providing health information. This is especially true of nurses involved in caring for people with cancer, due in part to the breadth of knowledge they require and accumulate when they are dealing with the implications of cancer. The education of the general public will be addressed in a later chapter (see chapter 3, The importance of communication and the provision of information in patient care) but it is important to point out that the public is made up of individuals each with their own unique background of beliefs and experiences born of and influenced by the culture and subculture to which they belong. Some of these people will develop cancer and it is their education by nurses that we wish to consider here.

This chapter will examine the principles of client education, and will provide guidelines to assist in the effective teaching of clients about the process and treatment of their disease and the opportunities for self-care. It is hoped that the strategies suggested for nurses will result in an increase in client knowledge and therefore greater client control. Research in the USA on effective education of clients affected by cancer (probably reflected in other English-speaking countries) indicates that initial negative experiences and beliefs give way to a practical realistic knowledge base, enhancing the ability of the client to:

- cope with the disease,

- reduce anxiety, and

- improve their self-concept and self-esteem (Bond et al., 1993).

# GETTING STARTED

The interaction between nurses and people with cancer or other chronic illness could be described as unique in that there is opportunity to form a bond and rapport that can last for years. Unlike most people who, when they are admitted to hospital, are sick, many people with cancer are admitted when they are well, albeit having recently been diagnosed with a potentially life-threatening illness. The nature of many of the current treatments for cancer is such that further admissions over ensuing months or years will be likely. The first meeting is, therefore, paramount in initiating a rapport that will last.

## How is this achieved?

The initial admission of the person with cancer signifies the beginning of a relationship between caregiver and client. The interaction should begin with an introduction and an orientation to the ward and ward processes (MacLeod, 1996). The logistics of these interactions are not always easy as the nurse is often occupied with other matters, but, ideally, time should be taken to make the person with cancer feel welcome and important.

There should be an area in the ward where the nurse can take the client and their family to discuss treatment and concerns without being overheard. This can encourage the client to speak frankly and can assist ultimately in making the client feel less vulnerable. The opportunity for questions to be asked and for the nurse to assess the client in a (relatively) private setting can complement the formal nursing assessment of physical and psychosocial aspects. Establishing a climate of reciprocal trust at this time can positively influence the client's stay on the ward, which must in turn lead to the client's being more receptive of information and support.

Despite a nurse's best efforts, however, there will be times when the client will not want to know about their treatment. Many people, even when they are healthy, rely on others to make major decisions. Such people often will not want to be personally active in their treatment choices (McCaffrey Boyle, 1997). When this occurs the oncology nurse must recognise and respect the right of the client *not* to know certain aspects of the disease and treatment. This can be difficult, and often conflicts with the goal of what the nurse is trying to achieve. Empowerment of and advocacy for clients are aspects of nursing practice that have received much attention and study; not to provide opportunities for the client to make their treatment choices would appear to conflict with this philosophy. By exercising their right *not* to know, the client is making a decision, and that decision should be respected.

## How is teaching carried out?

The teaching that takes place in the hospital (or home) environment can utilise several different techniques:

- programmed learning
- literature
- audiovisual materials
- personal instruction

### Programmed learning

This is a formal type of learning that sets out material in programmed sequential steps. This form of learning can be especially useful when familiarising people with tasks, for example, operating continuous infusion devices or Graseby pumps. The steps can be explained in written material or, as is becoming more common, with the use of computer packages or CD rom. Programs can be designed that test the knowledge of the participant, then direct them to multiple-choice questions. The program can acknowledge a correct answer or otherwise. The advantage of this type of learning is that it actively engages the participant, is often portable (allowing the material to be reinforced in the home environment) and is able to indicate a correct or incorrect response. There have been a number of such packages developed. Some have been produced by companies involved in the manufacturing of equipment; others have been designed by various disciplines of health professionals to assist in educating people on topics such as drug regimes and analgesic guidelines.

## Literature

The provision of literature is probably the most common form of supplying information to clients, but it is important to acknowledge that a brochure or booklet is useless unless people read it. It is incumbent on the nurse therefore not only to provide the literature, but also to ensure that it is readable, easy to interpret and 'client friendly' in its focus. The nurse should be there as a support and to answer queries. In Australia, most oncology units have information booklets and brochures covering a realm of topics, and the various state Anti-Cancer Councils are able also to provide information.

When devising such literature there are several factors that need to be taken into consideration including:

- readability;

- the type of font used (some fonts are more readable than others);

- the use of diagrams and pictures; and

- explanations of jargon.

Many clients who read this type of literature do not have scientific or medical backgrounds. Consequently, explanation in lay terms or with the use of diagrams is important. Topics such as an explanation of neutropenia lend themselves to the writer becoming very technical. The layperson will not concentrate on concepts that they cannot understand, so it is essential to keep the text simple and explain each concept in terminology that can be easily understood. A nurse should not assume, for example, that all clients will know what a 'cell' is. A simple explanation or diagram may be necessary.

An educational model used in the chemotherapy unit at the Peter MacCallum Cancer Institute involves a combination of written materials and visual aids, depending on what is being taught. Skills such as care of central lines can be learned readily with the use of a video. Additionally, an introductory booklet is given to the client and explained by the nurse prior to the client's first treatment. Writing space is provided in this booklet so that drugs can be listed, along with the client's regimen and chemotherapy schedule. The important points of the educational session are reinforced in discussions at subsequent admissions.

Although this structure for teaching and assessment appears fairly broad, it is easily individualised, depending on the client, and can be planned by the nurse according to the client's condition. This type of teaching gives the nurse, at each admission, the opportunity to assess the client's knowledge, skills, energy level and ability to concentrate. Issues such as anticipated length of stay and discharge planning can all be included in this type of educational session. An advantage of this type of teaching and learning is that the literature can be translated into different languages and, if necessary, interpreters can be employed to aid in communication.

## Audiovisual materials

As with programmed learning the use of audiovisual materials can be an effective way of getting messages across. Both commercially produced and 'in-house' videos of procedures showing what will happen when a client undergoes treatment allay much of the fear associated with the procedure. Video and audio cassettes can be loaned to the client to take home to study. In addition, these cassettes can be given to family and friends thereby accomplishing an educative role at the same time as allowing the family to appreciate what the client is experiencing. An advantage of this form of education is that it does not always require words so clients can see what occurs and gain some understanding no matter what language they speak. A well-filmed video may require little additional explanation.

Handing a client a video to take home does not guarantee that the client will understand what is being taught so it is very important that follow-up is conducted. This allows the opportunity to assess the effectiveness of the education. Clients should always be given a telephone number on which they can reach a resource person should any problems or queries arise.

## Personal instruction

Personal instruction can be given in two ways:

### 1.      *As a group*

Traditionally, nurses have conducted instructional antenatal classes or classes for people undergoing cardiac surgery and many other procedures. To run classes in the oncology setting is not difficult, but there are some inherent pitfalls.

With the field of oncology being so vast, it is easy to ignore the individual. The subject matter being taught to a group is not necessarily applicable to everyone in that group. A client undergoing radiotherapy for breast cancer, for example, may have many concerns different from those of someone undergoing radiotherapy for testicular cancer. Further concerns may arise when less-than-ideal group dynamics prevent people from raising concerns in the group situation. Providing time for the group to get to know each other and to interact can prevent such situations occurring (Murray et al., 1985).

The logistics of group education for people with cancer are not always easy, but the benefits can be great. For newly diagnosed people to meet other people who are cancer survivors can have a beneficial influence because they realise that not all people with cancer die. The opportunity to talk about treatments and to receive hints as to how to combat treatment side effects is vast.

### 2.      *Individually*

One-to-one instruction allows people to ask questions more easily. It also enables the nurse to question the client on individual areas of concern. In a recent study on educational needs of oncology clients, both clients and nurses reported that the one-to-one conversation was the most effective source of information about cancer (Griffiths and Leek, 1995). In some areas of cancer nursing, nurses can be somewhat reticent in asking appropriate questions and tackling certain subjects. Sometimes there is reason for this, but if client education is going to have the desired effect, that is, a gain in knowledge by the client that will aid in their self-care and enhance their ability to cope favourably with their disease, all areas must be dealt with.

For many nurses it is difficult to talk about certain issues, for example, sexual dysfunction or modification. This is especially true if there is an age or gender difference between the nurse and the client. Although this topic will be discussed in detail in a later chapter (see chapter 6, Cancer and sexuality — a neglected issue?), I am highlighting it here to tell a story against myself which demonstrates the importance of covering all aspects of a client's treatment. I was in my mid-thirties when this incident occurred, but it has stayed with me for many years, and I have never made the same mistake again.

*As a clinical consultant in chemotherapy, I was familiar with educating people prior to their treatment. One morning a gentleman in his late seventies was admitted with a haematological malignancy to have his first cycle of chemotherapy that morning. His elderly wife accompanied him.*

*As was my practice, I took them both aside, introduced myself, made a cup of tea and sat down and discussed aspects of the gentleman's treatment. The chemotherapy regime was CHOP (cyclophosphamide, doxorubicin, vincristine and prednisolone). A part of my spiel was to cover aspects of care of body fluids in the home, for example, flushing the toilet twice after each use. At this point the gentleman's wife asked if there was any danger to her. I explained that, as long as the precautions I outlined were followed, there would be none. She then said, 'No, I mean when we have sex.'*

*I confess that I was guilty of not covering the topic of sex in this instance. In retrospect I think I probably assumed that sex was not a priority to people in their late seventies. And who was I anyway, a 35-year old, to talk to a couple old enough to be my grandparents about their sex life?*

*Rather ashamedly I advised the use of a condom and talked openly to them about lethargy and just when they might have sex.*

*I was later to find out that the couple had been married for only two weeks!*

The lesson that I learned from this incident was to not assume anything when speaking to people about subjects of a personal nature. Where it is appropriate I now approach the subject of sexual effects and precautions with slight humour. For example I will say to an elderly woman, 'Now don't you go getting pregnant!' and wag my finger at her. The ladies always laugh, which allows me to become serious and say, 'No really, the nature of the drugs is such that . . . '. Making a joke allows me to raise the subject without either party being embarrassed.

With experience, each nurse will develop a teaching style that suits best. The styles will be many and varied and some will feel more comfortable than others. The overall aim, however, is to choose the style that is most appropriate for the individual or group being taught. For example, what works with the elderly might not be as useful with a group of children. With this in mind, it may be beneficial for nurses to review and trial other styles, even if these do not always feel as comfortable as the one the nurse–teacher is used to.

## CULTURAL AND SOCIAL ATTITUDES

Data from the United States has linked lower socioeconomic status and ethnicity to higher mortality rates of cancer, perhaps because of a negative attitude to cancer screening programs found among people in these categories. Some of the negative barriers identified are embarrassment, lack of confidence and lack of knowledge (Sugarek et al., 1988). This kind of negativity, coupled with the emotional distress of being diagnosed with cancer, can adversely affect people's capacity to learn. Grassman (1993) suggests that special consideration is required for people who are acutely ill, anxious or suffering discomfort. She claims that these factors can interfere with

> motivation to learn, and attention span, as well as with the learning
> process itself (Grassman, 1993:670).

It is paramount, therefore, for the nurse to attempt to make every client feel as comfortable and as much at ease as possible. Family members should always be involved unless there is some good reason why not, for example, the client's own wish or some cultural consideration (see chapter 15, Multiculturalism — implications for cancer care). When a nurse is dealing with someone who does not have a good command of English, the nurse should involve interpreters and try to be familiar with the customs of the culture to which the client belongs. Such procedures can only assist in the communication of knowledge.

## INSTILLING HOPE

> By providing emotional support, understanding and patient teaching
> about the disease and treatment, oncology nurses may enhance hope
> and desire for life within and among their patients and families
> (Hickey, 1986:133).

Clearly, to instill hope is the optimal goal of good client education. A realistic, genuine and caring attitude on the part of the nurse, honestly answering and anticipating questions, can all contribute to a positive outcome.

To maintain the 'hope status quo', that is, not to take hope away, can be much more beneficial than giving a client false hope. When educating a client about cancer and the treatment of cancer, it is easy to be falsely optimistic — and sometimes falsely pessimistic. To find the right balance takes practice and experience.

# CONCLUSION

Providing effective client education and relevant information has the potential to enhance the welfare and progress of people with cancer. The stress incurred when diagnosed with a potentially life-threatening disease can be great. Communication and efficient imparting of information is often a crucial factor in a client's treatment.

Oncology nurses are in an excellent position to pursue this important aspect of nursing and become providers of information that can benefit all health disciplines. There are future opportunities for nursing research to

- investigate teaching interventions,

- evaluate what is taught, and

- tailor new and innovative teaching methods.

The 1990s have often been described as the information age. Armed with information and adroit communication skills, oncology nurses are well situated to become the pivotal influence in the provision of client information and care into the twenty-first century.

## References

Bond Johnson J, Blumberg BD (1993): Teaching Strategies: Patient Education. In: Groenwald SL, Hansen Frogge M, Goodman M, Henke Yarbro C (1993): *Cancer Nursing: Principles and Practice.* Boston: Jones Bartlett.

Grassman D (1993): Development of inpatient oncology educational and support programs. *Oncology Nursing Forum* 20 4: 669–676.

Griffiths M, Leek C (1995): Patient education needs: Opinions of oncology nurses and their patients. *Oncology Nursing Forum* 22 1: 140.

Hickey SS (1986): Enabling hope. *Cancer Nursing* 9 3: 133–137.

MacLeod MJ (1996): *Practicing Nursing — Becoming Experienced.* New York: Churchill Livingston.

McCaffrey Boyle D (1997): Lecture to Nurses, Peter MacCallum Cancer Institute, Melbourne.

Murray R, Zetner J, McDowell P (1985): Health Promotion Strategies. In: *Nursing Assessment and Health Promotion Strategies Through the Life Span*. Norwalk: Appleton & Lange.

Nolan A (1995): Remaking the Nurse's Role. In: Nolan A and Hazelton L (1995): *The Practising Nurse*. Sydney: Saunders.

Public Health Association of Australia (Victorian Branch) (1997): *Images of Public Health*.

Sugarek NJ, Deyo RA, Holmes BC (1988): Locus of control and beliefs about cancer in a multi-ethnic clinic population. *Oncology Nursing Forum* 15 4: 481–486.

Swerissen H, Duckett S (1997): Health Policy and Financing. In Gardner H (1997): *Health Policy in Australia*. Melbourne: Oxford University Press.

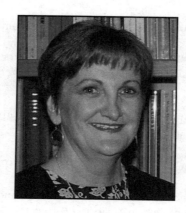

**SANCHIA ARANDA**
**Master of Nursing, Bachelor of Applied Science (Advanced Nursing),**
**Registered Nurse,**
**Member of the Royal College of Nursing, Australia**
**Associate Professor and Deputy Head of**
**the School of Postgraduate Nursing, The University of Melbourne, Australia**

Sanchia has worked in cancer and palliative care nursing since 1979 in both adult and paediatric settings. Sanchia originally trained as a nurse in New Zealand before moving to Australia in 1979. She did an oncology course at the Royal Marsden Hospital in London. In 1989 she developed the cancer/palliative care nursing course at La Trobe University in Melbourne and in 1996 developed this course for delivery in distance mode. In March 1997 Sanchia took up the position of Associate Professor in Palliative Care, a joint appointment between The University of Melbourne's Centre for Palliative Care and School of Postgraduate Nursing. Sanchia is a board member of the International Society of Nurses in Cancer Care, a position that has provided her with a wonderful opportunity to view Australian nursing within the wider global context.

# Chapter 2

## *Challenges and opportunities — educating the nurse for cancer care*

## INTRODUCTION

Cancer is the second leading cause of death in Western countries, including Australia and the USA. It is predicted to become the leading cause of death by the year 2000 as a result of the continued aging of the population and the decline in deaths from cardiovascular disease. All nurses, regardless of their area of practice, are likely to confront the health needs of people with cancer. Most will also experience cancer at personal or family levels or be called upon to offer advice or support to friends and relatives affected by cancer.

The preparation of nurses for cancer care is an important aspect of the social response to cancer. Cancer nursing education is a broad, multifaceted field of endeavour, occurring at several levels within the education system as well as in practice settings. Following a brief historical overview, this chapter focuses on the challenges and opportunities that exist in the formal preparation of nurses for cancer care. The chapter draws on my experience in developing and teaching the cancer nursing course at La Trobe University from 1990 to 1996. The final section of the paper offers potential students a guide to choosing a postgraduate course.

## A BRIEF HISTORY

Cancer emerged as a specialist field of health care practice in the 20th century. During the second half of the 19th century cancer treatment centred around surgery, with patients receiving care in general surgical units. Modern nursing was at an early stage of development, with schools of nursing being established in most major Western cities. The charge nurse was usually a trained nurse, however, students provided most of the direct care to patients. Cancer was understood as incurable, with a death rate of 90 per cent (Yarbro, 1996).

The development of radiotherapy in the first half of the 20th century increased attention on the possibility of curing cancer. Later developments in systemic chemotherapy treatment and improved understanding of cancer biology improved the overall approach to cancer treatment. By the 1960s the field of oncological medicine had come of age. Treatment of cancer was no longer futile, with one in three people alive five years after their cancer diagnosis.

Cancer nursing as a specialisation underwent parallel development with medical oncology. In the 1950s several countries established specialist education programs. In 1950 the National Cancer Institute in the USA ran a three-week course for 30 nurse educators and pilot cancer nursing programs commenced around the country (Yarbro, 1996). A year-long cancer nursing internship for foreign nurses was offered by Memorial Hospital and New York University. Similar developments occurred in the United Kingdom. The Royal Marsden Hospital began a 113-hour course in the early 1950s with major curriculum review taking place in 1958. The new course commenced in 1961 with 12 students, three of whom were from overseas. The four weeks of study were spread over six months but the course was not professionally recognised until after the establishment of the Joint Board of Clinical Nursing Studies. In 1974 the Royal Marsden became the first hospital to gain course approval from the Board (Brian Lake, personal communication). The Peter MacCallum Cancer Institute (PMCI) in Melbourne, Australia, commenced its radiotherapy nursing course in 1958. This later evolved into a broader course and was retitled the Oncological Nursing Course in 1976 and later the Cancer Nursing Course (Lois Gorman, personal communication).

The rise of cancer as an area of specialist practice in both medicine and nursing has resulted in an enormous body of professional knowledge. Cancer nursing education between the 1950s and the 1980s focused on providing for the needs of people receiving cancer treatment. During the 1990s roles in cancer nursing have evolved and diversified. Improvements in survival have resulted in cancer survivors who have specific and often unrecognised rehabilitation needs. Developments in cancer control, through prevention and early detection, provide alternate roles in cancer care. Knowledge developments in care of the dying, arising out of the hospice movement, are also an essential part of modern cancer care. Cancer care nursing, while still retaining a focus on treatment-related care, now encompasses nursing roles in a range of settings and with diverse groups of clients. Genetic counselling, bio- and gene-therapies and the dramatic shift to ambulatory care are just some of the emerging opportunities for nurses.

Nursing itself has undergone a revolution and the emerging body of nursing knowledge must be integrated into the learning of nurses in cancer care.

Narrow and limited perspectives of cancer nursing education, centring on treatment-related care, will not prepare nurses for the roles demanded of them. The information explosion means that, as our radius of knowledge grows, so the circumference of the unknown expands. The future of expanding knowledge and increasing care complexity demands a lifelong approach to professional education. Nurses require education that prepares them to practice creatively in changing environments and from multiple perspectives.

# UNDERGRADUATE EDUCATION IN CANCER NURSING

In Australia all undergraduate preparation of general registered nurses occurs in the tertiary sector. While there are considerable advantages for students through degree preparation as entry to practice, the rapidly expanding knowledge base in nursing cannot be taught in three academic years. Undergraduate nursing providers face a very real dilemma — how to prepare practitioners for diverse practice settings within a curriculum that cannot focus on specialist practice.

The Australian approach to this dilemma has been to develop national nursing competencies that set the minimum standard of practice expected of a new graduate. The competencies are broad and require specific development and application in the area of practice selected by the graduate. There is minimal room within the undergraduate curriculum for specialist education of any kind. The fact that cancer is a common health problem ensures that the majority of student nurses care for people with cancer during their undergraduate experience. However, given the extent of the problem, should cancer care specialists pressure for specific cancer focus within the curriculum? Is it possible to dispel myths and negative attitudes towards cancer without a specific focus on cancer care? McCorkle, Preston and Volker (1996) argue that it is crucial during nursing training to dispel myths and create positive attitudes to cancer and the people affected by it.

One approach to the problem has been the appointment of 10 American Cancer Society Professors of Oncology Nursing across the USA. These leaders in the specialisation, while largely teaching at master's degree level, also oversee the cancer content of undergraduate curricula. This approach targets cancer care expertise into the development and teaching of generalist topics such as ethics, communication skills and the provision of comfort measures. Recently, the Professors have attempted to influence curriculum development in more direct ways by recommending cancer content for undergraduate courses (Sarna and McCorkle, 1995). The core concepts identified are extensive (Table 2.1) and indicate a move away from the idea of generalist competencies. The four-year curriculum in the USA offers greater scope for the inclusion of specialist content than the Australian three-year curriculum.

## Table 2.1 Curriculum and self-study guide for core concepts in cancer nursing

I.  What is cancer?
    Historical perspectives of cancer
    Current status of cancer as chronic
        illness
    Carcinogenesis (basis of initiation and
        promotion, acquired genetic
        aberrations)
    Alterations in cells (e.g. cell cycle)
    Immunosuppression and cancer
    Differentiation of benign and malignant
        tumours
    Tumour classification
    Invasion and metastasis
II. Cancer prevention: risk reduction
    Primary prevention: assessment of
        individual risk factors, assessment
        of exposure to carcinogens, family
        history
        Tobacco prevention/cessation
        Sun exposure
        Diet and weight control
        Occupational exposure
        Older age as risk factor
III. Early detection of cancer (secondary
        prevention)
    Cancer epidemiology: international,
        national and local perspectives;
        differences by age, gender,
        socioeconomics, racial/ethnic
        group; incidence, prevalence and
        death rates
    Screening guidelines
    Relationship of early detection to
        decreased morbidity and mortality
    Early signs and symptoms of cancer
    Self-detection methods
IV. Principles of cancer diagnosis and
        treatment
    Importance of tissue diagnosis
    Principles of a staging workup (and
        TNM classification)
    Common sites of metastasis
    Purposes of treatment
        Curative, palliative, adjuvant,
        neo-adjuvant

Basic principles of action: risks/benefits
    Chemotherapy
    Radiation therapy
    Surgery
    Biological response modifiers
    Bone marrow and stem cell
        transplantation
    Adjuvant and neo-adjuvant treatment
V.  Nurses' role in resolving ethical issues
        and dilemmas
    Treatment decision-making
    Informed consent/clinical trials
    Issues in palliative care
    Shift from cure to palliative therapy
    Questionable methods
VI. Symptom management
    Common side effects of treatment and
        tumours, especially
        pain
        infection/fever
        bleeding
        nausea/vomiting
        cachexia/anorexia
VII. Psychosocial aspects of cancer care
    Trajectory of coping with cancer as
        chronic illness across life span and
        in different populations
    Patient and family psychosocial
        responses
    Sexuality
VIII. Continuum of care
    Economics and politics of care: access,
        quality of care and outcome
    Rehabilitation: living with cancer and
        lifestyle changes
    Referral to psychosocial resources
IX. Occupational/safety and emotional
        concerns for caregiver
    Radiation precautions
    Risk of infection/isolation precautions
    Occupational exposure to
        chemotherapy agents
    Coping with grief and loss
    Emotional burnout

(Reprinted with permission of Lippincott-Raven Publishers)

The dilemma of preparing nurses to care for people with cancer within a generalist framework remains. My assumption is that specialist practice arises from the application of generic nursing skills and a strong foundation of knowledge around a specific client group — in this case, those affected by or at risk of cancer. Two questions arise from this assumption that should drive attempts to influence undergraduate curricula: which of the generic skills are most applicable to cancer care and what elements of cancer content are necessary to develop a beginning application of these skills to cancer care?

Defining the relationship between core competencies in nursing and skills in cancer care is an important challenge. Specialist cancer care nurses must consider this relationship and determine those aspects of cancer care that are core requirements of all graduate nurses. The inclusion of specialist cancer care nurses as associate staff of university schools of nursing could assist with a consideration of this issue and in influencing curriculum development. Such nurses could provide current clinical cases for class discussion, offer curriculum advice and be involved as sessional lecturers.

The provision of undergraduate student placements in cancer care areas is a further area of concern for many university schools of nursing. Specialist areas often resist student placements, while continuing to voice concerns about the quality of graduates. Improvements to cancer care require a committed approach to the preparation of undergraduate nurses from specialist settings. It is useful to view students of nursing as potential recruits to the specialisation. Clinical placements are opportunities to excite and stimulate interest in the specialisation and a source of staff recruitment. Positive student experiences in cancer care will translate to graduates better able to care for people with cancer.

## POSTGRADUATE CANCER NURSING COURSES

Specialist nursing education has a strong tradition in Australia. Hospital schools of nursing provided the greatest proportion of specialist education, such as certificate courses, until the late 1980s. Most of these certificate courses became courses in the university sector at graduate certificate and graduate diploma levels. This move was both a logical next step following the transfer of undergraduate nursing and a consequence of economic pressures within the health sector.

The Peter MacCallum Cancer Nursing Course ended in 1991. This was a time of rapid expansion of specialist postgraduate diplomas in the tertiary sector. The first Australian tertiary cancer nursing course began at La Trobe University in 1990. Similar courses are now widely available across Australia. During the same period economic issues became central to health management. Nursing education was an expensive luxury to some hospital administrators. Nurse educators employed in hospitals became an endangered species as downsizing and redundancies became the focus of the 1990s. The rapid shift of courses in all nursing specialisations from hospitals to universities failed to take account of the broad status of nursing education. Most nurses, having trained in the hospital system, felt ill-equipped to undertake specialist education within the university sector and disenfranchised by the changes. In addition, there were few educators left in the hospitals to help them overcome the perceived barriers to undertaking tertiary education.

The decision to re-establish the Peter MacCallum Cancer Nursing course in 1997 occurred in the context of three existing tertiary-based courses in Melbourne. The course's re-emergence disrupts the wholesale move of postgraduate nursing to the tertiary sector and highlights the uneasy relationship between university and health sectors in relation to nursing education. At least two key areas of difference lie at the heart of this uneasy relationship — clinical performance and course content.

# CLINICAL PERFORMANCE

Hospital certificate courses aimed to prepare nurses for specialist practice. However, in addition to staff development, these courses were a useful means of staff recruitment. The courses offered students the opportunity of paid and supervised employment in combination with theoretical learning while also meeting the hospital's service needs. Rotation through various departments of the hospital exposed students to a range of clinical experiences while also preparing a flexible work force for the hospital. Clinical skills were linked closely to course achievement and students were closely supervised in practice. The synergy of this relationship between learning and practice utility has been central to the development of specialist nursing in Australia.

The movement of hospital courses into the tertiary sector, with few exceptions, broke this close relationship between theory and practice. While university courses offered students study opportunities that did not put their current employment at risk, this was offset by reduced opportunities for student rotation and supervision of clinical practice. At La Trobe University, students in the early years of the course were often experienced cancer nurses studying to gain formal recognition of their experience. Clinical supervision of these students raised little concern as they had vast experience that enhanced their classroom learning. Over time the student group changed to be younger and more inexperienced, requiring greater attention to clinical learning. As a tertiary educator, I found theoretical concepts harder to teach in the context of minimal clinical experience and course funding did not provide for extensive supervision of practice.

# COURSE CONTENT

In contrast, university programs generally offer students a greater range of course content than hospital courses. Hospital-based curricula must take account of the tension between student learning needs and hospital service requirements. In my own experience, courses in England had an overemphasis on medical management of specific diseases and treatments. This focus helped to ensure patients were 'nursed' according to hospital procedures. The focus on particular cancer nursing knowledge and skills was minimal.

University courses in cancer nursing facilitate a shift in focus from medicine to nursing. In addition to traditional disease-focused care, attention is placed on specific nursing content. Nursing skills in translating medical information, educating patients and families, providing support and managing unpleasant symptoms become central to role development. In addition, greater opportunities to explore nursing roles outside the hospital allow a focus on cancer prevention, community education, home care, survivorship and the terminally ill. University courses also give students the opportunity to combine their studies with other areas of interest. Nurses in cancer care, gerontics and home-based palliative care come to understand the similarities in their practice as they spend time in shared classes. These opportunities expand networking and ultimately lead to better outcomes. The emphasis on research within the university sector is also important given current demands to demonstrate effectiveness in health care.

The balance of clinical to theoretical learning and the utility of course content to practice are important areas of concern. Other areas of concern include entry requirements, articulation of courses and recognition of prior learning. To maximise student learning in each of these areas improvements are needed in communication and collaboration. However, emphasis on resolving these issues must not occur at the expense of a consideration of the future learning needs of nurses in cancer care. Concentration on the site and content of learning will not prepare nurses for future cancer care.

Core curricula in cancer care attempt to set the parameters of practice in cancer care. Possibly the Oncology Nursing Society's core curriculum is the best known (Ziegfeld, 1987; Clark and McGee, 1992). Core curricula are comprehensive and incorporate a broad range of nursing content in addition to treatment and disease information. However, the basic assumption of all core curricula is that all nurses in cancer care require the same information. Credentialling activities associated with core curricula attest to this and seek to ensure standardised levels of knowledge within the cancer care nursing community. These efforts reproduce the tension between student needs and service requirements present in past and current systems of preparing nurses for cancer care. While core curricula help to ensure standards of practice in treatment and disease-related care, most offer little to prepare nurses for the rapidly changing health care environment.

## THE FUTURE

In 1994 Debi Boyle and colleagues published an important series of articles on the future of cancer care (Boyle et al., 1994a, 1994b; Boyle, 1994; Engelking, 1994; Harvey, 1994). In this series the authors predict the future profile of people receiving cancer care services, the nature of those services and the treatments likely to exist. Ambulatory care, targeted treatments and advanced technology, a vulnerable aging population and increased consumer demands for effective services are just some of the predictions made. Nurses of the future, while retaining an important direct care role, will also supervise the practice of an expanding network of support workers; a new and uncharted aspect of nursing practice. The shift to ambulatory and home-based care gives renewed emphasis to the nurse's role in client and caregiver education. Teaching responsibility will include establishing outcome measures that demonstrate this learning (Liebman, 1997).

Boyle and her colleagues (Boyle, 1994; Engelking, 1994; Harvey, 1994) produced a number of futuristic job advertisements that hint at the roles nurses concerned with cancer care may undertake (see examples in Table 2.2). Any reading of these potential roles cannot fail but demonstrate the enormous gap between current educational focus and the likely reality of future practice. Advanced practice, creativity, role-boundary breakdown, information technology and flexible work practices are just some of the challenges facing nursing educators.

Boyle (1994) argues that current perspectives on nursing education will shift to a greater emphasis on preparation in the clinical environment. While this may sound like a return to hospital courses, perhaps it also reflects the growing emphasis on preparing students for meaningful roles in their workplace. Short courses with high flexibility to meet an immediate workplace need, delivered in and specific to that environment, will be demanded. Fixed curricula will have little place as the information and technology explosions break down barriers and demand lifelong approaches to learning. Preparation for advanced practice will take on greater emphasis as increasing chronicity and complexity forces new approaches to care. These approaches will need to be outcome effective and cost effective, and increasingly delivered in the home environment. The site of education will change as information technologies promote the shift of university learning to the workplace. Opportunities to undertake courses globally, across a range of universities and other education sectors, will force greater flexibility on traditional providers.

The current separation of nursing specialties will blur. It is not difficult to imagine nurses with joint preparation in aged, cancer and palliative care working in local communities to provide a comprehensive service for complex clients. Perhaps more difficult to grasp is the likely blurring of role delineation between currently established disciplines. Many of the future roles in Table 2.2 are not discipline specific and expose preparation challenges that negate a predominantly nondiscipline-based approach to education. In many ways the generalist education of nurses at the undergraduate level ideally prepares them to undertake postgraduate preparation in these futuristic roles. However, postgraduate education will need to feature flexible and role-focused learning rather than content if nursing is to take a central role in shaping and managing the future of cancer care.

### Table 2.2 Opportunities in the 21st century

**WANTED: PATIENT-READINESS EVALUATOR** to work in a partnership with a group of medical oncologists in a large, university-affiliated bone-marrow transplantation (BMT) program. Responsible for conducting pre-transplant patient/family screening to determine resources and deficits of each BMT candidate. Also devises plan to bolster patient/family reserves and readiness for the procedure, communicates the plan to nursing staff, and follows patients through the process and for an extended post-transplant period.

**WANTED: MINORITY NEEDS SPECIALIST** to coordinate the Latino Cervical Cancer Awareness Project, with offices in Dallas and Houston. This model program was developed by three Texas oncology nurses to address the reality that Hispanics account for 48 per cent of all cervical cancer deaths in their state. Responsibilities include worksite education, patient advocacy during the statewide multimedia broadcast of tumor boards, and creation of ethnically customized educational programs and television specials about cervical cancer and other gynecologic malignancies.

**WANTED: CANCER RISK COUNSELOR/SCHOOL NURSE** at the Brookwood Elementary School. This person will provide intensive cancer prevention education to children and their parents. Responsibilities include home visits to evaluate and counsel high-risk families

**WANTED: COST-BENEFIT ANALYST** to work jointly with the financial and patient care services departments of the Community Health Network in Santa Fe, NM, to analyse the quality/cost relationship of specific procedures and interventions.

**WANTED: TREATMENT OPTIONS ADVISOR** for a 36-bed cancer research unit for which policy mandates consensus sessions involving the prescribing physician, the patient, and family members as a prerequisite for the transcription of orders to initiate new therapies. The successful candidate is an oncology nurse with a background in clinical trials and demonstrated coalition-building skills. Responsibilities include arranging family conferences; participating in treatment recommendation sessions; serving as a liaison among patients, families, nurses, and physicians; and serving as a member of a bioethics committee.

**WANTED: GERO-ONCOLOGY INTENSIVIST NURSE** who is a graduate of the Cross-Training Program of Norris Cancer Center/University of Southern California or Moffitt Cancer Center/University of South Florida. (In the late 1990s, these were the first federally funded programs to cross-train advanced practice nurses in oncology, gerontology, and critical care in the home setting.)

Adapted from Boyle, 1994; Engelking, 1994; and Harvey, 1994

# CAREER PLANNING AND GRADUATE EDUCATION

## Client-focused practice

Given this future scenario, how can a nurse interested in a cancer care career best prepare for the opportunities that will arise? Building a career that focuses on a specific client group may be one possibility. Traditionally nursing careers have been built around existing roles, such as the day centre chemotherapy nurse. The steps in role preparation have been focused on treatments and skills established as being used by these nurses, such as cannulation. Each nurse is prepared to fit into an existing model of practice, with little consideration of the changing face of client care or cancer management. A career focus built around a client group can help to widen this understanding. Questions about how clients cope with the shift to home care and about who will care for them at home arise more readily from a client-focused approach to role development. The nurse needs to spend some time considering the skills required to work with this specific group of clients, both now and in the future. Once the nurse identifies the knowledge and skills required, informed choices about education can follow.

## Choosing a graduate course

A graduate education can open career opportunities. Graduate preparation at the master's degree level is essential for those nurses seeking advanced practice roles. Hagopian and McCorkle's 1993 paper on choosing a master's degree program in the USA is a useful starting point. Although written within a traditional approach to education and cancer care practice, it offers some worthwhile points applicable to the Australian situation.

Perhaps the most important starting point is to identify the target audience of the course. Is it aimed at beginning, intermediate or advanced practitioners? Where there is a mixed skill group, what opportunities exist to work at a faster pace than other students? What are the aims of the course in terms of student outcomes? Are the aims in keeping with personal learning goals? Obtaining a match between student and course is the first step in obtaining a successful education experience.

Hagopian and McCorkle (1993) suggest exploring the resources of the school with whom you are planning to study. It is important to view the concept of resources broadly and not just in terms of library facilities, computing facilities and other environmental issues. Those who anticipate changing employment or social circumstances should ask about the flexibility of learning environment. Is the course available off campus or by contract learning? What relationships exist between the university and clinical environments that might provide additional learning sites? Are there staff with appropriate expertise in the areas you wish to study?

The curriculum is obviously a key area requiring consideration by the student. Questions about the curriculum and about previous student work will help to expose the level of flexibility and creativity of the course. Students may have specific goals for learning that are not part of the set curriculum. Therefore it is important to identify the possibilities for elective studies or for substituting other subjects for those set for the course. Where elective studies are available, students should explore the potential barriers to taking these, such as additional fees, timetabling and student quotas for popular courses. Talking to students who have undertaken the course in previous years is a good way of finding out the strengths and weaknesses of a specific course.

Assessment is closely linked to curriculum issues. Potential students should ask questions about the assessment tasks expected. To what extent do assessment tasks allow topic flexibility and relate meaningfully to the student's work environment? Assessments that can link to the student's work environment are more likely to provide opportunities for employer support. Does all assessment fall at the end of semester? A spread of assessment across the semester offers the opportunity for early feedback about progress and decreases the potential for overload.

The strength of research teaching in the course is a major area of concern as demonstration of clinical effectiveness becomes a health service requirement. Many students complain that they study the same research content at varying university levels. Asking questions about research teaching, the level of focus on clinically relevant issues and expectations for skill development will help to identify those courses offering the best research preparation. At master's degree level it is also important to ask about completion rates as these indicate how far the course prepares students for success. It is also important to identify potential research/thesis supervisors. Matching student to staff member in this area is crucial to research success. Students should look for a breadth of methodological interest amongst staff rather than focus solely on expertise in cancer care. Examining the publications of prospective supervisors can help to identify areas of similar interest and concern and can assist in predicting potential areas of conflict due to competing perspectives.

## CONCLUSION

This chapter, above all, emphasises a considered and critical approach to education in cancer care. The rapidly changing health environment and the exploding knowledge base around cancer provide the context for cancer care education. Our modern world has few truths and little security, health care being no exception. Those who will contribute most to cancer care are those who deal with this uncertainty with flexibility and creativity. Educational programs in cancer care must offer skills for lifelong learning and must harness the creative energies of students. While there needs to be some level of standard education for cancer care this must not occur at the expense of diverse student outcomes and innovative approaches.

# References

Boyle DM, Engelking C, Harvey C (1994a): Making a difference in the 21st century: Are oncology nurses ready? *Oncology Nursing Forum* 21 1: 53–55.

Boyle DM, Engelking C, Harvey C (1994b): Taking command of the future: Getting ready NOW for the 21st century. *Oncology Nursing Forum* 21 1: 77–79.

Boyle DM (1994): New identities: The changing profile of patients with cancer, their families, and their professional caregivers. *Oncology Nursing Forum* 21 1: 55–61.

Clark J, McGee R (eds) (1992): *Oncology Nursing Society Core Curriculum for Oncology Nursing* (2nd edn). Philadelphia: W.B. Saunders Company.

Engelking C (1994): New approaches: Innovations in cancer prevention, diagnosis, treatment and support. *Oncology Nursing Forum* 21 1: 62–71.

Hagopian GA, McCorkle R (1993): Choosing a master's program in cancer nursing in the United States. *Oncology Nursing Forum* 16 6: 473–478.

Harvey C (1994): New systems: The restructuring of cancer care delivery and economics. *Oncology Nursing Forum* 21 1: 72–77.

Liebman M (1997): The right to know. *Clinical Journal of Oncology Nursing* 1 3: 59

McCorkle R, Preston F, Volker DL (1996): Cancer Nursing Education Today. In: McCorkle R, Grant M, Frank-Stromborg M, Baird S (eds): *Cancer Nursing. A Comprehensive Textbook* (2nd edn). Philadelphia: W.B. Saunders Company.

Sarna L, McCorkle R (1996): A cancer nursing curriculum guide for baccalaureate nursing education. *Cancer Nursing* 18 6: 445–451.

Yarbro CH (1996): The History of Cancer Nursing. In: McCorkle R, Grant M, Frank-Stromborg M, Baird S (eds): *Cancer Nursing. A Comprehensive Textbook* (2nd edn). Philadelphia: W.B. Saunders Company.

Ziegfeld CR (ed.) (1987): *Oncology Nursing Society Core Curriculum for Oncology Nursing.* Philadelphia: W.B. Saunders Company.

# Personal communications

Lois Gorman, Director of Nursing Education, Peter MacCallum Cancer Institute, Melbourne, Australia.

Brian Lake, Director of Education, Royal Marsden Hospital, London, England.

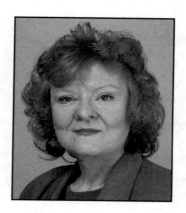

**DOREEN AKKERMAN**
**Bachelor of Science, Helen M. Schutt Trust Fellow***
**Director, Cancer Information and Support Service, Anti-Cancer Council of Victoria,**
**Australia**

Doreen has more than 25 years' experience in community and professional education and, through her work as a Senior Research Associate in Oregon in the USA and as Director of the Cancer Information and Support Service (CISS) in Victoria, 15 years in the design and implementation of comprehensive information services. She has supervised CISS in Victoria since January 1990, designing and developing the model which, in 1994, was voted the Australian model for cancer information and support.

Doreen led the Cancer Information Service Short Course at the World Conference for Cancer Organisations in Melbourne in March 1996 and, together with Christy Thomsen from the National Cancer Institute, USA, and Catherine Dickens, from BACUP in the United Kingdom, established the International Cancer Information Service Group under the auspices of the International Union against Cancer (UICC).

Doreen is committed to establishing information and support services and to the exchange of skills, information and tools in order to provide units of excellence which may assist in decreasing the impact of cancer on people's lives.

*The Helen M. Schutt Trust is an Investors Philanthropic Trust set up in Victoria, to assist with health provision. Doreen received a $250 000 scholarship from the Trust to help with CISS (Victoria).*

# Chapter 3

## *The importance of communication and the provision of information in patient care*

### DIFFERENT PATIENT NEEDS A NURSE SHOULD BE AWARE OF

Whilst the ideal source of information for a patient is their treating doctor, a patient often goes into shock when first given a cancer diagnosis, so they may not fully comprehend what their doctor is saying. Patients often feel inhibited about requesting clarification and information regarding their diagnosis and condition at a level that they can understand.

A small percentage of people do not want to know too much detail about their disease as they prefer to put their total trust in their doctor and treating team. There is a delicate balance between being provided with enough information to make informed decisions about treatment and having the right not to be bombarded with a lot of information one does not want. The health professional, however, should always be aware of giving the patient the choice (Fallowfield et al., 1995).

In many cultures, any discussion regarding a person's illness and treatment is made with family members initially and then with the patient, or with selected members of the family group present at the time of consultation (Norman, 1996). Nurses should be aware of the cultural mores of patients under their care and endeavour to comply with what is acceptable practice in those cultures without compromising the rights of the patient, and in the light of legal and ethical issues in Australian health practice.

# HOW CAN A NURSE MEET INDIVIDUAL NEEDS?

The most trusting and intimate relationship that a patient develops when regularly visiting a clinic or day treatment centre or during a stay in hospital is with the nurse. The nurse provides physical care, comfort and frequent contact. The nurse is often the first person with whom a patient or a member of their family will tentatively raise a question. Therefore it is vitally important that, as caring health professionals, nurses ensure that they have up-to-date, credible information and skills regarding the following:

- legal and ethical issues concerning provision of information and treatment;

- the psychological impact of cancer and treatment upon the patient and family;

- the importance of communicating effectively and providing psychosocial support to people affected by cancer;

- cultural mores for different ethnic groups regarding cancer and treatment;

- understanding and management of symptoms arising from cancer and its treatment;

- information on appropriate support programs and resources available for people affected by cancer; and

- the issues of loss and grief relating to a diagnosis of cancer.

In this chapter, the impact of various stages of cancer upon the patient will be explored, together with the appropriate level of information required at each stage and ways of providing information and referral to appropriate resources in order to help the patient and their family to cope.

It is important to also recognise stress in oneself and colleagues and to be able to take advantage of opportunities to share information with the multidisciplinary team in order to enhance team performance. There are simple ways of helping each other to reduce the impact of stress. Reducing the team's level of stress enables the team to provide optimum health care to others.

# GUIDELINES AND PROTOCOLS

Each medical centre/hospital has protocols for the provision of information to patients and their family, and all health professionals should be aware of the guidelines and protocols in their place of work. They should also be aware of legal liability regarding the provision of information and duty of care.

# DIAGNOSIS

Once a person hears that they have a cancer diagnosis, their life changes forever. They may experience myriad feelings — anger, grief, frustration, disbelief — all at once, with fear of death being the most common, overriding response (Sussman, 1995).

Callers to the Cancer Helpline at the Anti-Cancer Council of Victoria have said that after the doctor told them they had cancer, they could not recall another word. One 'came to' hours later, wandering around a major department store and could not remember getting there. It may take days, weeks or months for a person to completely absorb the full meaning and impact of cancer upon their lives.

## SETTING THE SCENE

People should always receive news regarding their diagnosis in a 'face-to-face' situation and they should be given the choice of having a friend or relative present (Sardell and Trierweiler, 1993). A longer-than-usual appointment should be arranged when the news to be given to the patient is 'bad news'. A nurse should be present during the consultation, especially if the patient is unaccompanied. It is good clinical practice to tape-record the consultation in which a doctor gives a cancer diagnosis to a patient. This tape can then be played over and over for the patient and family at home.

It is important for nurses working in a clinic setting where people are given cancer diagnoses to check that the person is not in shock before they leave the clinic. A quiet place should be provided for all who receive a cancer diagnosis to sit for a while and the nurse should check that they have a safe way of getting home. If possible, some close family member or friend should be available to provide comfort and support.

Before the patient leaves, an early appointment should be made to meet with the doctor for a follow-up consultation within the next week or as soon as possible after that. This will give the patient time to absorb what was said during the diagnostic consultation and discuss it with family and friends and will provide them with the chance to address any issues or concerns that arise.

Patients have told the Cancer Helpline that they really appreciated doctors who, at the disclosure of their diagnosis, stressed each patient's individuality and how cancer affects different people in different ways. They have said that this enabled them to foster hope, see their illness as a challenge and build up ways of facing and 'fighting' their disease.

Before the patient leaves, they should be offered a telephone number at the clinic to call, if they have any further questions, or be provided with the Cancer Helpline brochure and the telephone number 13 11 20 (Australia wide) for them to contact for adjuvant information and support.

# AT THE START OF TREATMENT

The patient and their family expect 'state-of-the-art' treatment and care from their clinician and hospital. They expect the health care team to be up to date with the latest in cancer research, information and technology.

Nurses working in the wards at a hospital may find their first contact with the cancer patient occurring after the patient has been through weeks of investigations and worry. The patient may be admitted to the ward for surgery or treatment, still unsure of what the outcome will be and in a state of confusion, grief, fear, anger and alarm.

They may be in awe of the clinician and the hospital setting, which is strange and intimidating. The nurse who welcomes them and assists them to settle into bed and place their personal belongings close by is seen as an ally and a person on a level to be trusted.

The nurse will provide information regarding what will happen during treatment, and ways of coping with any side effects that may occur and concerns that may arise. The nurse also monitors the patient's progress and builds up rapport whilst assisting the patient with basic hygiene and day-to-day procedures. This forms an excellent foundation for future communication. The nurse may translate, in a logical, comprehensive way, medical 'jargon' that a patient does not understand and also may act as an advocate and point of referral within the multidisciplinary team.

# DURING ACTIVE TREATMENT

From time to time, as treatment progresses, the patient must be given the opportunity to ask questions. This can be done either formally or informally. However, when a patient or a member of their family asks questions regarding their cancer and treatment, only their specific questions should be addressed. For example, it is inappropriate at the point of diagnosis to overwhelm a patient with information regarding secondary or metastatic cancer.

Nurses can offer to obtain for patients written information that they can read at their own pace and discuss with their doctor. There is also a support booklet called *Life with Cancer* (available in all Australian states) which discusses the emotions a cancer diagnosis arouses, how to tell friends and family and ways of coping. If there is either a Living with Cancer education program, a cancer support group or an oncology social worker at the hospital, the patient should be provided with information and a contact number.

It is wise to be aware that every word a nurse speaks is often taken as the ultimate, expert source of medical advice. A casual remark made about taking vitamins may be regarded as a compulsory prescription by an anxious patient or their family. The nurse should be comfortable with saying in answer to some questions: 'That is not my area of expertise, you should discuss that with your doctor' or 'That is something I am not familiar with, but I will find out for you'. The promise should always be followed up and the information or referral contact provided.

Each person has individual needs, but people who are newly diagnosed with cancer require basic information regarding:

- the specific type of cancer;
- how that type of cancer is treated;
- why that treatment is used;
- what the treatment consists of and how it will be given;
- ways of coping with the side effects of the treatment; and
- information regarding supportive care.

This information may have to be provided in small amounts, talking with the patient over a period of one or two days to ensure that they can understand, absorb and process the information provided.

During treatment a patient will often turn to the nurse for instructions regarding:

- what symptoms to look out for and be concerned about;
- what to do about mouth care;
- where to obtain literature regarding nutrition and diet; and/or
- referral to appropriate support services, for example, the dietitian, oncology social worker, rehabilitation services, and pastoral services.

The nurse, through the provision of good information and quality referral, helps the patient to retain quality of life and to keep their life as normal as it can be during the active treatment phase.

Concerns may arise about fertility, sexuality and sexual practices which may be affected by disease or treatment. The nurse is often the first person who is asked what to do. The nurse should answer any questions honestly and in a nonjudgmental manner. A nurse who does not know the answer to any question should say so, but should always follow up and find out not only the information the patient requires but also an appropriate health provider to address the issues raised.

Confidentiality is fundamental to all nursing practice, and information regarding the patient's personal details should not be released, even to another health care professional, without the patient's permission.

It is often a good idea when making an appointment for adjuvant treatment to have a booklet available for the patient that explains the treatment. In Australia state cancer councils produce booklets regarding specific types of cancer and guides for understanding chemotherapy and radiotherapy. These booklets are free and are distributed to hospitals on a regular basis. Many hospitals also produce their own fact sheets for patients. These sheets may also be obtained by calling the Cancer Helpline at 13 11 20 from anywhere in Australia.

# CLINICAL TRIALS

Written information is available clearly outlining specific/relevant information for individual trials. This information is written by the hospital and drug company conducting the trial. Before a trial is initiated the protocols, and all issues concerning the trial, are discussed and approved by an ethics committee.

Explanation about clinical trials invariably exposes some uncertainty about treatment and the need for ongoing research into treatment outcomes. Clinical trial participants, therefore, need a complete range of information regarding the clinical trial, the length of the trial, drugs and protocol being used, and any side effects that may be expected. Clinical trial patients will have much more contact with the clinical nurse specialists attached to the trial and must have enough information and support to make informed decisions at any phase of the trial. This includes the ability to drop out of the trial at any point.

# REMISSION

Although patients may have found attending treatment on a regular basis difficult (it may have encroached on their lifestyle), they often feel abandoned at the completion of treatment. When told that they now do not need to come in as often, and an appointment is made for a couple of months hence, they often feel lost. They will no longer have that contact with the nurse and other members of the team who cared for them, who chatted with them and asked about how they felt. They have often built up a rapport with other patients and so they are left to their own resources.

When talking with the patient at the final appointment for treatment the nurse can provide them with a contact number in case they feel the need to contact the clinic and at this point may link them in with a patient support program or cancer support group being run at the hospital or out in the community. Groups for cancer survivors are now starting to evolve in Australia as the number of people 'living with cancer' continues to grow.

# RECURRENCE

People who experience a recurrence of cancer say that the 'second time around' comes as more of a shock and is often accompanied by a feeling of despair and devastation as they realise that this cancer is not going to go away. They often feel extreme anger as they have been doing everything they were supposed to do and the cancer has still come back.

At this time a patient will often face their own mortality and the nurse should offer the opportunity for them to talk about their feelings.

Northouse and Northouse (1996) state that:

> The single most important problem confronting cancer patients is loss of control — a feeling of powerlessness resulting from the inability to predict or have an impact on events surrounding the illness.

> Patients who are communicated with and treated in predictable ways will feel more competent about how they are handling their illness. Allowing a patient to communicate with the same nurse over the course of illness, is one way of enhancing the patient's sense of control.

People often associate palliative care with death and do not realise the benefits related to pain and symptom control during each phase of the cancer journey. Pain may be tolerated because of a reluctance to 'bother' the nursing staff or because of the association of the use of opiates with drug addiction. The nurse can allay these fears and explain the importance of controlling pain and symptoms in order to gain quality of life. The nurse should monitor the patient's level of pain and, if pain or symptoms are an issue, refer the patient to the palliative care team within the hospital.

It is important to discuss the fact that even if the cancer cannot be cured it is often possible to manage and control it for a considerable length of time. There are support booklets available called *Coping with Advanced Cancer* and *Caring for the Person with Advanced Cancer*. The nurse can give these to the patient and their carers.

# SIGNS TO BE AWARE OF

People dealing with a cancer recurrence may become severely depressed. The nurse should be aware of this and look for signs of depression or an inability to cope such as insomnia, loss of appetite etc. and should bring this to the attention of the treating doctor and multidisciplinary team. The patient may then be referred for individual assessment, counselling and appropriate medication.

At this time, people often benefit from a visit from a member of the pastoral care team, if religion and spirituality have been a part of their lifestyle. Non-Christian religions are well represented in Australia and a rabbi, imam or other religious minister should be available if required.

There are many hospice and palliative care programs throughout Australia offering both at-home and in-patient care. Patients, carers or family members may refer themselves to a hospice or palliative care organisation. Respite care is also provided by health care facilities or volunteers in order to give the carer a break. There are carers' associations that provide information packets, telephone advice, assistance and linkage with carers' support groups.

Information on how to access these services may not be available as a matter of course at the hospital. The nurse needs to be aware of all resources that offer these services and, if necessary, link the patient and their family directly to the service.

# TERMINAL PHASE

Rituals which surround dying and death differ in many cultures; who is told, when they are told and who should be present when the information is given is strictly circumscribed in many cultures.

Australian ethical standards must be adhered to in the provision of terminal care, but acknowledgment and attention to cultural mores is important, so the nurse should be aware of what is appropriate for the person being cared for.

Many people find facing the closure of their life extremely difficult. When treatments fail or there is a decision made to discontinue treatment and the person becomes more ill and more fragile, both family and patient need a lot of information and support.

Every opportunity should be given for the patient to discuss their feelings at any time during this phase of care. There is no 'right' way or scheduled 'proper pathway' for dying. Each individual finds their own way and although this may not be the way we, as nurses, would choose, we owe it to the patient to respect their wishes and provide care and support for them until the moment of death.

Listening is vitally important — just being there as a witness, listening and holding a hand can be of tremendous support and may be the specific type of support that is required. The nurse needs to acknowledge symptoms and relieve them, and should do this without a sense of fuss. Because we may not have been able to provide a solution to every problem does not mean that we have not been of help.

Provision should be made to give the patient and family privacy and space, so that they can be together, although the nurse should be available to the family to answer any questions. Hospice and palliative care services offer psychological support to patient and families alike and Grief Line offers anonymous loss and grief telephone counselling. There are bereavement counsellors and bereavement support groups which are available for family and friends.

Nurses may find it helpful to use their own multidisciplinary team meeting to discuss their feelings after the death of a patient and to link in with their informal support group if a psychologist is not available for debriefing and support for the team and staff members.

# MAKING THE MOST OF THE MULTIDISCIPLINARY TEAM

The nurse, as the member of the multidisciplinary team who has the most contact with the patient, can:

- provide necessary information for care coordination;
- act as an advocate for the patient; and
- provide the most detailed information regarding the patient's wellbeing.

A multidisciplinary team that works well recognises the value and contribution of all members. It enables optimum coordination and delivery of care for the patient and should be a source of support for all members. If a peer support program is not in place at the hospital or other place of work, nurses may want to consider setting up a primary nursing 'buddy system'. Two or three nurses may agree to be each other's source of emotional support when the stress of dealing every day with people affected by cancer at all stages seems overwhelming.

The support nurses may telephone each other and meet in an informal way, on a regular basis to debrief about their work. They provide each other with nonjudgmental opportunities to talk over problems and concerns, to talk about grief and loss which nurses deal with on a daily basis.

Walking, jogging, dancing, swimming and listening to music are all excellent ways of reducing stress. Nurses should find out which works best for them and, either alone or with a friend, build that activity regularly into their lives. Those who find that stress still continues to be a problem should seek professional counselling.

Where a hospital or clinic does not have team meetings or a health professional support group in place, nurses should advocate for one to be developed. It is important for nurses to set in place for themselves ways of dealing with stress so that they may remain functioning and 'meeting the challenge' in what continues to be an extremely demanding but ever-rewarding role in the provision of health care to people affected by cancer.

# SPECIALISED NURSE COUNSELLING ROLES

The role of nurses is ever expanding and changing and those working in specific areas have developed specialised skills, for example,

- breast care nurses,

- nurse counsellors working on a cancer help line, and

- nurses working in stomal therapy.

## Breast care nurses

The Anti-Cancer Council of Victoria Breast Cancer Support Service has had trained breast cancer support nurses in hospitals throughout Victoria since 1975. In 1997 a unique course was designed for the accreditation of breast care nurses. Nurses successfully completing the course will expand their skills for providing information and support to women through the whole continuum of the breast cancer journey from diagnosis to death. The National Breast Cancer Centre has also funded a pilot project in four Australian collaborating care centres to develop and test a new expanded role for Australian breast care nurses as part of the multidisciplinary care team.

## Cancer nurse counsellors

National cancer information services throughout Australia, Canada and Singapore are based on the model of the Anti-Cancer Council of Victoria. Registered nurses with oncology qualifications and experience provide telephone information and support to people affected by cancer, and to their family and friends. The nurses discuss specific types of cancer, treatment options, psychological support etc. and send written information to the caller.

## Stomal therapists

Nurses who complete a specific stomal therapists' course can specialise in the provision of one-to-one information and support to people with an ostomy. The nurses provide pre- and post-operative counselling for the patient and the family, after-care of the patient and ongoing review of their physical and psychological condition.

# CONCLUSION

This chapter, in reviewing the importance of communication and information in the provision of patient care, has demonstrated also the importance of the nurse's role in such provision. The value of the nurse–patient relationship can never be overestimated and, as a source of information and support, the nurse is irreplaceable.

# References

Fallowfield L, Fordi S, Lewis Shon (1995): No news is not good news: Information preferences of patients with cancer. *Psycho-oncology* 4: 197–202.

Norman Catherine (1996): Breaking bad news: Consultations with ethnic communities. *Australian Family Physician* 25 10, October: 1583–1587.

Northouse LL, Northouse PG (1996): Interpersonal Communication Systems. In: McCorkle R, Grant M, Frank-Stromborg M and Baird S (eds): *Cancer Nursing: A Comprehensive Textbook* (2nd edn). Philadelphia: W.B. Saunders Company, pp. 1211–1222.

Sardell AN, Trierweiler SJ (1993): Disclosing the cancer diagnosis: Procedures that influence patient hopefulness. *CANCER*, December 1, Vol. 72, No. 11.

Sussman N (1995): Reactions of patients to the diagnosis and treatment of cancer. *Anti-Cancer Drugs* 6 Supp. 1: 4–8.

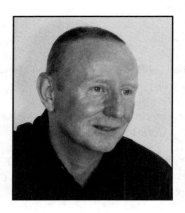

**GORDON POULTON**
**Graduate Certificate in Advanced Nursing Cancer/Palliative Care Nursing,**
**Certificate in Cancer Nursing, Registered Nurse,**
**Member of the Royal College of Nursing, Australia**
**Nurse Educator, Peter MacCallum Cancer Institute, Melbourne, Australia**

Gordon began his nursing career in 1979, and has worked predominantly in oncology since commencing employment at the Peter MacCallum Cancer Institute in 1980 as a State Enrolled Nurse. After completing his General Nursing Training at Box Hill Hospital in Melbourne in 1985, Gordon returned to the Cancer Institute where he has been involved in a variety of cancer care areas. Following the completion of a Certificate in Cancer Nursing at the Institute in 1988, Gordon worked for six years as a Clinical Nurse Consultant in the chemotherapy unit. During this time he was given the responsibility of coordinating the pilot Hospital in the Home program, and participating in both the clinical and academic aspects of chemotherapy nurse education.

Gordon has presented at numerous forums at local, national and international levels on topics ranging from nutrition in immunocompromised persons to informed consent in people undergoing clinical trials. He is a past convenor of the Victorian AIDS Council (VAC) Nurses Group and deputy convenor of the VAC Support Group. At present he is completing a Master of Health Science in Cancer Nursing at Victoria University of Technology in Melbourne. Gordon's private life is devoted to socialising with his friends, listening to a wide variety of music and tackling cryptic crosswords.

# Chapter 4

## *Breaking bad news*

Nurses working in the cancer setting are often confronted with situations in which they must communicate bad news. This arduous aspect of the cancer nurse's role can be fraught with stress and anxiety which can in turn be deflected to the client. It is imperative, therefore, that communication skills be taught as early as possible in a student's training and they should be taught not only to students of nursing but to everyone who is studying to be a health professional of any kind (Franks, 1997).

Parathian and Taylor (1993) suggest that communication is an important aspect of nursing curriculum, but that *effective* communication comes with practice and experience. This chapter will examine the art of communication in nursing, focusing in particular on the nurse's role in the breaking of bad news

## WHAT IS BAD NEWS, AND HOW DO NURSES KNOW WHEN THEY ARE COMMUNICATING IT?

Deciding whether news is good or bad can often be a subjective judgement. What may seem bad news to the communicator may be good news to the person receiving the news. For example, telling someone that their discharge will be delayed because they require a blood transfusion due to anaemia resulting from recent chemotherapy may well be better news than explaining to someone that they can go home because their tests do not show any reason for their recent lethargy and dizzy spells.

Franks (1997:61) defines bad news as
>    any news that drastically and negatively alters the patient's view of her or his future.

She emphasises that bad news is not necessarily related just to topics of death and dying or issues around incurable illness, and that in fact there may be a number of reasons that make news bad for a particular person at a particular time.

The *Nursing Times* Professional Development Supplement (1994:5) describes bad news as

> drastic changes, either real or potential, in the quality of life or the ending of hope of an improvement, again real or imagined, for the future.

The extent of the bad news will often influence the decision as to who conveys it. Traditionally, bad news surrounding death and dying has been conveyed to clients by medical staff, and is often incorporated into a conversation when results of investigations are being reported. When this occurs there is often a support person on hand to be with the client, usually a relative or friend, but it can be whomever the client wishes to be present (Faulkner et al., 1994). Franks (1997) acknowledges that, of all health professionals, nurses spend the most time with the client, and that there is a heavy emphasis in nursing education on communication so nurses may well be the best-equipped health professionals to break bad news. Franks argues, however, that the breaking of bad news should not be the domain of nurses alone; doctors and other health professionals cannot totally abrogate this often unpleasant task. Nevertheless, the role of breaking bad news is part of the work of a nurse and this chapter sets out to help nurses to hone their skills in this aspect of the job.

## A PROCESS

Faulkner et al. (1994) suggest that the art of breaking bad news is a skill that is achieved through practice and experience. They set out a collection of strategies that form a definitive process both for breaking bad news and for handling the effects of bad news and they present it as a flow chart. Figures 4.1 and 4.2 are adapted from the flow chart.

(Figures 4.1 and 4.2 are adapted from Faulkner A. et al., Breaking bad news — a flow diagram. *Palliative Medicine* 1994; 8:145–51. Reproduced with permission of the publishers.)

## Figure 4.1 Breaking bad news

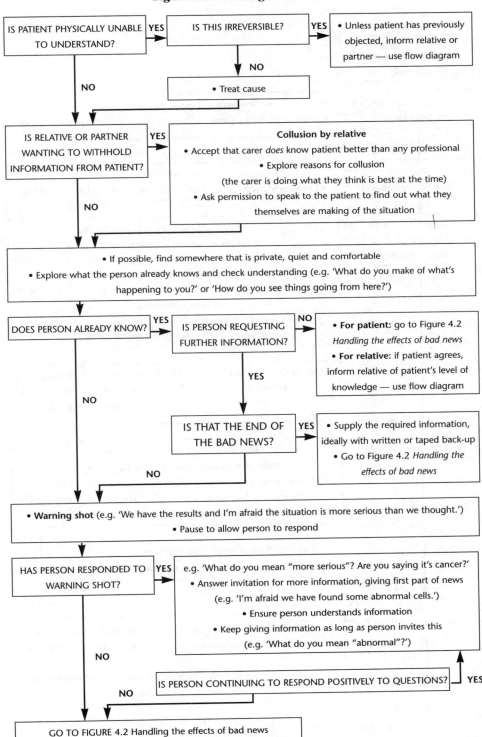

## Figure 4.2 Handling the effects of bad news

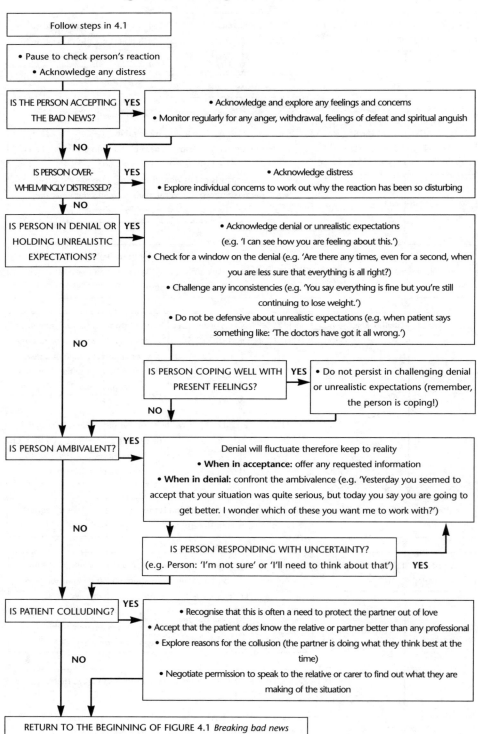

# THE IMPACT OF BAD NEWS

There are many factors that can influence the impact of bad news including:

- prior information;
- the demeanor of the communicator;
- the physical environment;
- the words used;
- the time taken to convey the information; and
- barriers in communication.

## Prior information

How much the client knows or suspects will have an influence on how bad news is received. If the client suspects a bad outcome, they may (sometimes unconsciously) have prepared themselves already for the news. This can often make the task of breaking the news less stressful for the nurse. Taking the time to find out how much the client knows is important when choosing the appropriate method of imparting the information. Prior experience with and knowledge of the client can help. For example, even a simple procedure such as a lumbar puncture or bone marrow biopsy may come as bad news and cause pain and fear in a person who has had previous bad experience with such procedures.

## The demeanor of the communicator

Body language can send powerful messages. Facial expression and voice tone can all help prepare people to receive bad news. Faulkner et al. (1994) suggest that preparation should include some sort of 'warning shot' (see Figure 4.1). In their article they give the example of opening the front door to a policeman in uniform. This situation often means bad news, but the police uniform acts as a warning shot and prepares the person. Nurses do not have this advantage with their uniform and instead must use words, actions and body language as their warning shot.

## The physical environment

Buckman (1992) suggests that if the physical setting is right, both the person breaking the news and the recipient of the news feel more assured and relaxed. Faulkner et al. (1994) imply that privacy is paramount, and that the optimal situation is a private room where all parties can sit down. For nurses working in a hospital setting where an interview room is not always available, screening the bed and sitting in close proximity to the client can at least give the illusion of privacy. The act of screening the bed also provides the warning shot and if the bed is screened reaction to the news is shielded from other people in the room, saving embarrassment to both the person to whom the news is conveyed and others in the room.

Ideally interviews should not be conducted standing up, although as Buckman points out, this is sometimes unavoidable. If the conversation is conducted standing up, Buckman says, then body stance is important. Standing closer to the person than you would normally reduces the opportunity of being separated by passers-by, and leaning against a wall can give the illusion that the you are not rushed.

While the scenario of a separate interview room with comfortable chairs and copious amounts of time for explanation and questions is the ideal, in reality this can be difficult to achieve. Moreover, such formal measures may not always be appropriate. Nurses are in the unenviable position that *any* information they convey may well be bad news. This can range from explaining to people reasons why their discharge is delayed to informing people that a loved one has died. While time and privacy are desirable for the latter, they are hardly essential to the former.

## The words used

There is no easy way to convey bad news to people, and choosing the appropriate words is difficult. However, to not convey messages adequately and correctly is to do a disservice to the client, and puts the nurse in a vulnerable situation.

It is important to remember that many 'lay' people will not understand medical jargon, therefore simple language is required. Indeed, even when information is put in lay, terms people fail to retain up to 50 per cent of what is said to them (Buckman, 1992). For this reason information should be given in small 'digestible' chunks, on the understanding that only parts will be retained, and that most will need to be reiterated at a later time.

## The time taken to convey the information

Bad news is, unfortunately, important news, so time should be taken both to convey the message clearly and to support the client during and after the message is conveyed. It is essential that the nurse listens for the concerns of the client and answers questions honestly and as best they can. It is better to admit that you are unsure of an answer than to answer either incorrectly or inadequately.

Payne and Walker (1996) hold that clients rarely ask questions if they do not understand what is being communicated because they are afraid of wasting the nurse's time and because they do not wish to appear foolish. Consequently the onus is on the nurse to convey news and information accurately and effectively, and to make certain that the information has been understood.

# Barriers in communication

There are many barriers that can block the effective communication of bad news. One of the major barriers is fear. This fear can be on the part of both the recipient of the news and the communicator of the news. Fear on the part of the recipient is a fairly common reaction. It is fear of an uncertain future. In a situation such as this the communicator can support the client by:

- allowing them to speak of their fears;

- reassuring them on any positive aspects of the news; and

- listening to their anxieties.

It is important not to take away all hope (Buckman, 1992; Franks, 1997).

Fear on the part of the nurse is one of the factors cited by Franks (1997) in the difficulty of breaking bad news. Franks claims that the nurse feels concern and fear that they will be blamed for the news. Further, there is a fear of upsetting or hurting —and therefore failing — the client. The uncertainty as to how a client will react and the feeling of helplessness in the communicator to cope with this reaction make the breaking of bad news an unenviable task. This is certainly one reason why we as nurses fear breaking bad news, but there are others including:

- fear of facing death ourselves;

- fear of eliciting an adverse or unpleasant reaction from the client;

- fear of admitting that we don't know the answers; and

- fear of expressing our own emotions.

Buckman (1992) claims that recognising these factors all help the nurse in overcoming the fear.


## REACTIONS TO BAD NEWS

> I became angry. Angry with the doctors. Angry with my family. And angry that life had dealt such a blow to Ron (Joyce, 1993:109).

Reactions from recipients of bad news are very individual, but many describe feelings of anger and helplessness (Joyce, 1993; Janet, 1993; Carole, 1993). How these emotions manifest will vary. Events and experiences that have evolved over years will influence individual responses. In some cases it is culturally appropriate for a recipient of bad news to become demonstrative when upset. In other cultures the opposite can happen and people can appear to become introverted and withdrawn.

Buckman (1992) describes disbelief as a common response, and suggests that this is quite normal. He claims that it is not up to the nurse to try to change the reaction, but merely to support the client and/or the significant others while they are experiencing the emotion. Nurses are not privy to the past experiences of many of their clients and therefore cannot predict their reaction. It is, however, the response of the nurse that will determine whether the client (or the client's family) will feel supported and cared for.

## CARING FOR OURSELVES

As cancer nurses we practice in an area of nursing that is conducive to a rapport being formed that can be very strong. It is conceivable, therefore, that we are often breaking bad news to someone who has become a friend. This can influence our emotions and play havoc with our psyche, so it is important that members of the health team have an outlet, somewhere that might be called the 'screaming room'. You can share the screaming room with someone if you wish, but primarily it is a place for you to let off steam, to cry if you want to, but to come to terms with this aspect of our work. A screaming room is not necessarily a physical place, although for many it is. (Traditionally, the hospital pan room has often been used as a physical screaming room for nurses, though for many it is too public). The screaming room may well be an emotional or spiritual place that can be accessed in a variety of ways, ranging from visualisation to meditation. I am not going to dwell on what or where, or even if, the screaming room has to be a physical place (caring for yourself and for your colleagues is covered in chapter 13, Caregiver support) but I do want to emphasise that it must exist.

## CONCLUSION

This chapter has highlighted some of the concerns of nurses dealing with the sensitive area of breaking bad news. Although suggestions have been made as to a process that might be followed, we must use our skills as nurses to determine what is most appropriate in any given situation. There is no one right way to break bad news but there are strategies to help us avoid doing it badly. Breaking bad news is not a pleasant task, but with experience, tact and compassion for both the client and ourselves, the task can be done and it can be done with minimal impact.

## References

Buckman R (1992): *How To Break Bad News – A Guide for Health Care Professionals*. Baltimore: John Hopkins University Press.

Carole (1993): Carole. In: Baxandall S, Reddy P: *The Courage To Care: The Impact of Cancer on the Family*. Melbourne: David Lovell Publishing.

Faulkner A, Maguire P, Regnard C (1994): Breaking bad news — a flow diagram. *Palliative Medicine* 8: 145–151.

Franks A (1997): Breaking bad news and the challenge of communication. *European Journal of Palliative Care* 4 2: 61–65.

Janet (1993): Janet. In: Baxandall S, Reddy P: *The Courage To Care: The Impact of Cancer on the Family.* Melbourne: David Lovell Publishing.

Joyce (1993): Joyce. In: Baxandall S, Reddy P: *The Courage To Care: The Impact of Cancer on the Family.* Melbourne: David Lovell Publishing.

*Nursing Times* Professional Development Supplement (1994): Breaking bad news: Knowledge for practice. 90 10, March: 1–8.

Parathian AR, Taylor F (1993): Can we insulate trainee nurses from exposure to bad practice? A study of role play in communicating bad news to patients. *Journal of Advanced Nursing* 18 5: 801–807.

Payne S, Walker J (1996): *Psychology for Nurses and the Caring Professions.* Buckingham: Open University Press.

# SECTION TWO

## *Tears and fears: The impact of the diagnosis*

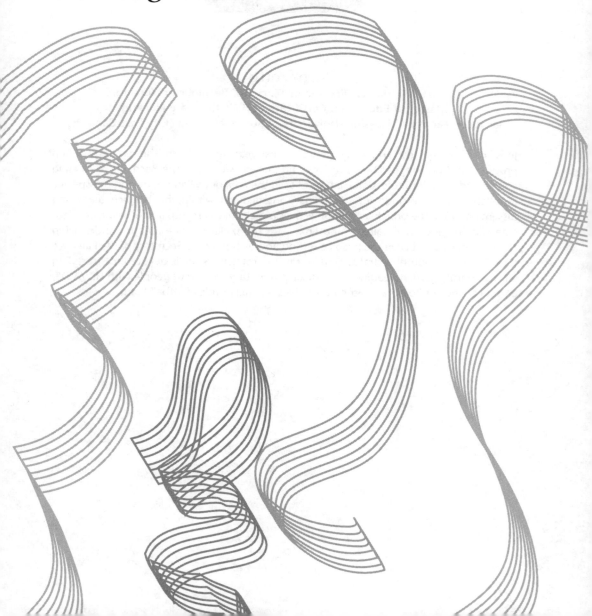

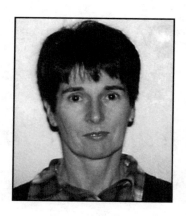

**JUDY ZOLLO**
**Registered Nurse, Diploma of Teaching, Bachelor of Nursing,**
**Master of Education, Certificate of Palliative Care Nursing**
**Lecturer, Faculty of Nursing, University of South Australia (City East Campus)**

Judy divides her teaching time between first-year students in the pre-registration program and post-registration students undertaking studies in the Bachelor of Nursing course. Judy's major professional interest lies in the area of palliative care and her specific research interests include interdisciplinary interactions within the hospice team and dissemination of the principles and objectives of palliative care into acute- and extended-care settings. Judy maintains strong links with the palliative care area by undertaking regular faculty practice in the hospice setting and by her role as Secretary of the Palliative Care Council of South Australia. Time out from professional life is devoted to struggling with an unruly garden, reading, undertaking voluntary work with people with HIV/AIDS, and following the fortunes of the Port Power Australian rules football team.

# Chapter 5

## *Hope — the inner strength*

## INTRODUCTION

Despite major advances in cancer therapies in recent years, malignant neoplasms remain a leading cause of death in our society. A diagnosis of cancer generates a range of responses, including fear, anxiety, treatment-related discomfort, anticipation of bodily disfigurement, and existential uncertainty (Herth, 1989:67). Counterbalancing this somewhat pessimistic outlook, De Vita reminds us that 'cancers, as a group, are among the most curable of chronic diseases' (cited by Hickey, 1986:133). Even when hopes for a cure are slim, Fryback (1993) notes that many individuals diagnosed with cancer have a period of time when they pick up their lives again and continue living without any significant degree of impairment. In contrast to patients who succumb to the physical and psychological stressors imposed by a diagnosis of cancer, those who pick themselves up confront, and, on some occasions, overcome the stressors (Post-White et al., 1996). Whilst a proportion of successful outcomes could be attributed to improved cancer therapies, the question of what contributes to clinically significant changes in cancer patients is far more complex, and not so easily answered (Rustoen, 1995). An equally important and increasingly recognised factor in some cancer cures may be the phenomenon of hope. Among nurses and other health care professionals, there is a particular interest in the physical and psychological value of hope to individuals suffering from a range of chronic or life-threatening illnesses. More specifically, increased attention has been given to examining the phenomenon of hope in patients with metastatic cancer (Yates, 1993).

51

# THE MEANING OF HOPE

Although attempts to accurately analyse and document the clinical impact of a concept as complex as hope are often preceded by attempts to define the concept, a precise definition of hope remains elusive. Although hope is seen as universal (Hinds, 1988) there is certainly no universal meaning for this multifaceted phenomenon (Herth, 1990). A similar notion is articulated by Frankl (cited by O'Connor et al., 1990), who sees the desire to give life purpose or meaning as the primary motivational force in humankind. This universal search for meaning, incorporating the concept of hope, is, however, unique and specific to each individual at the level of observable behaviours, attitudes and beliefs. A final comment on the difficulties encountered in refining a definition of hope is provided by Fromm (cited by Hall, 1990:179), who attributes difficulties in understanding the precise nature of hope to its being

> so integral to humanness that it is difficult to describe in words. It is like a fish trying to understand the meaning of water.

The difficulties in conceptualising and operationalising the concept of hope are reflected in the fact that specific definitions of hope are almost as numerous as articles and studies devoted to this concept. The following selection of definitions represents only a small number of those presented in the literature. Rather than formulating her own definition, Fryback (1992:150) presents definitions from a range of authors, who describe hope as:

- a multidimensional life force marked by a confident yet uncertain expectation of achieving a future good which, to the hoping person, is realistically possible and personally significant (Dufault and Martocchio, 1985);

- a state consisting of anticipation of a continued good, an improvement, or the lessening of something unpleasant (Miller and Powers, 1988); and

- a belief in the existence of a positive future (Hinds, 1988).

In the specific context of terminal illness, Herth (1990:1256) sees hope as

> an inner power that facilitates the transcendence of the present situation and movement toward new awareness and enrichment of being.

Finally, Raleigh (1992:443) cites Stotland, who defines hope as

> an expectation of goal attainment modified by the importance of the goal and the probability of attaining it.

Although this range of definitions emphasises the idiosyncratic nature of hope, the crucial contribution of hope to human survival provides a point of agreement for several authors. These include Bolander (1994), who considers hope essential to the search for meaning in life-threatening illness, and Hall (1990), who suggests that hope is so vital to life that its loss is equated with loss of life itself. Fryback (1993:150) supports this view that hope is essential to life with Seigel's declaration that 'refusal to hope is nothing more than a decision to die', while Simsen (1988), in a similar pronouncement, states that without hope we begin to die. Further commonalities arising from the many definitions of hope can also be found. Nowotny (1989:58) is just one of a number of authors to identify several similar critical attributes for the concept of hope, including the following:

- hope is future oriented;
- hope includes active involvement by the individual;
- hope comes from within a person and is related to trust;
- hope relates to or involves other people or a higher being; and
- the outcome of hope is important to the individual.

## IS HOPE THE ESSENTIAL KEY TO SURVIVAL?

However hope is defined, it has been recognised increasingly as an important factor in the long-term survival prospects of those with cancer. For many individuals, a diagnosis of cancer is viewed initially as a threat because it throws into sharp focus the fact that the future is now far less certain. It is at this point that some individuals mobilise their energy to actively fight the threat posed by their diagnosis. A key weapon in this fight is hope. Rustoen (1995) suggests that, although not normally present at a conscious level, hope is propelled into the consciousness by the crisis of receiving a cancer diagnosis and is manifested as a belief that the present situation can be modified, and a way can be found out of the difficulties. This conscious decision to fight cancer with hope would include, for many, hope for a cure or hope of a longer life. While difficulties exist in proving unequivocally a direct causal relationship between high levels of hope and an apparent cure or long-term survival following diagnosis of cancer, can it be claimed with any more certainty that such outcomes are the result of modern cancer therapies, a range of complementary therapies, a visit to a religious shrine, or mere serendipity? Findings from an increasing number of studies of hope as an element in the human response to life-threatening illness offer some support to the view that this phenomenon may positively influence survival outcomes for some individuals.

Hickey (1986:133) suggests that in the newly diagnosed cancer patient, a strong desire for life, supported by hope, 'can act as a powerful stimulus for living', and that the hopeful may realise their hopes simply by striving actively toward the goal of survival. In a study of the struggle by terminally ill individuals to maintain hope, Herth (1989) demonstrates a significant relationship between high levels of hope and effective coping with the physical, sociological, and psychlogical stresses of a cancer diagnosis and subsequent treatment. In discussion related to this study Herth states that coping effectively while undergoing chemotherapy may influence the effectiveness of therapy, and that effective coping is dependent upon a range of variables, including hope.

Poncar (1994:34) supports her statement that 'a positive relationship between hope and survival has been determined' by citing results from two studies:

- Greer found that breast cancer patients with highly optimistic attitudes survived much longer than those who 'responded with stoic acceptance or feelings of helplessness or hopelessness' (cited by Poncar, 1994:34); and

- Christman suggested that hopefulness was 'associated with better psychosocial adjustment in cancer patients receiving radiotherapy for cure or control of their disease' (cited by Poncar, 1994:34).

Hinds (1988:79) advances the claim that
> hopefulness is believed to directly influence health and illness states
> by helping individuals to maintain, regain, or augment health.

In support of this claim, Hinds cites the suggestion by Gottschalk that cancer patients identified as energised by hopefulness are likely to have better outcomes, before concluding that
> hopefulness may function as both biological and psychological
> response modifier, thereby influencing tumour progression and sense
> of well-being in cancer patients (Hinds, 1988:79).

Finally Rustoen (1995:359) puts forward her perspective on the role of hope in directly improving health outcomes of people with cancer by referring to Sims's suggestion that
> the ability to see a situation as hopeful improves psychological
> adjustment and may influence survival.

Perhaps better than any of the authors already referred to, Hall (1990) demonstrates the link between hope and improved survival outcomes for patients with cancer. Hall adds a particularly poignant touch to a study of the struggle by diagnosed terminally ill persons to maintain hope as she describes her own diagnosis of metastatic cancer seven years prior to carrying out the study. Her experiences have led to her conclusion that hope does play a role in the survival of individuals with a potentially fatal diagnosis, and that 'hope is something all people need until they take their last breath' (Hall, 1990:178). Hall's interviews with 11 men with stage two HIV disease, and her experiences in dealing with issues of her own mortality, provide the backdrop for her claims on behalf of the power of hope. Some of the anecdotes related by Hall are particularly powerful, including this tale from one interviewee:
> I finally realised that AIDS was just one possible way of meeting your
> death. So I repeated over and over to myself, 'Shot by an irate
> Iranian, crashing in an airplane, being killed in a car wreck, being
> shot at random by a passing bullet', and started just statistic counting,
> and came to the honest to God realisation that my chances of being
> killed while walking down Sixth Street were statistically greater than
> dying of AIDS in the next five years. That little tidbit of information
> was all that I needed to push it a little bit further out of my reality. In
> this way, I learned to manage my destiny, circumstances, and
> situation (Hall,1990:182)

Ten of Hall's 11 interviewees related similar tales of maintaining a positive outlook by using 'affect-control' strategies, or strategies to control the emotions. Establishing a future and maintaining a positive outlook on life was vitally important to these men, all of whom reported high levels of hope for the future. This hope can be seen in some of the following statements:

- *It came to me all of a sudden that all it takes is just you dealing with the needed changes. I have transformed the shame into pride about the things that I can accomplish, and the effectiveness of my state of mind has helped some others that I know.*

- *I am an optimist. I think my spiritual and mental makeup has not been studied or given credence to. I am not real pleased with what the doctor told me, but I did not panic. I have a determination to enjoy life, even though I don't have everything I would like to have*

- *I would tell others to change their attitude and outlook. Don't accept a death sentence. Don't feel like a victim. You can live with it. You can cope with it.*

In stark contrast to these ten interviewees, most of whom reported feeling healthier mentally, physically, and spiritually than ever before, was the one interviewee who did not visualise himself as having a future life on earth, and who did not have a structured self-care regime worked out. He died within eight months, although Hall, who was with him when he died, saw him as choosing to 'focus his hope on life after death' rather than as bereft of hope (Hall, 1990:183). What is significant about this example is Hall's suggestion that, just as the presence of high levels of hope may positively influence survival and life quality in persons with potentially fatal illnesses, absence of hope may have the reverse effect.

Along with the majority of her interviewees, Hall describes herself as just one more person with a potentially terminal condition who has experienced the process of losing and then regaining hope. Her relatively long-term survival with metastatic cancer, her extensive reading on the subject of hope, and her investigation of the phenomenon of hope in other seriously ill persons has led her to the view that

> life is hope, and that hope, in our culture, is an orientation toward the future that must be maintained in every stage of life, regardless of one's degree of frailty or the potential hazards of an uncertain future (Hall 1990:180).

One of the key ideas highlighted by Hall and her interviewees is that in a society where medical labelling has such a powerful and pervasive effect on our views of reality, maintaining hope is not always easy. In addition to mounting a struggle against their disease, those diagnosed with cancer face a fight against those who would 'remove all their anchors and thus force them into an unknown future' (Hall, 1990:180). Fryback (1993) also comments on the destruction of hope by a medical care system which, in setting artificial time limits, assists such predictions to become self-fulfilling prophecies. Although medicine, with its advanced knowledge and understanding of disease stages, may rob some terminally diagnosed persons of hope, there are others who deal with these scientific predictions, by seeing them 'as a challenge in order not to lose hope' (Fryback, 1993:179).

I well remember such a person in my own practice. This 94-year-old patient had been admitted to a hospice for pain assessment and to give his elderly carer a well-earned respite. As this was the first time I had met this gentlemen, I was keen to build up an accurate picture of his emotional, psychological, and spiritual health in order to determine what his needs might be during this admission and following discharge. I had been led to believe that his condition was terminal, so asked, as gently as I could, how he had coped so far with his diagnosis, and how he thought he and his carer would manage following discharge. He proceeded to tell me that he had every intention of being around for a good while longer, and that when he had received his original diagnosis more than 10 years previously he had consciously chosen to treat the predictions of his doctors as a challenge to be met and overcome, rather than having the decency to succumb quietly as his doctors obviously expected him to. His determined struggle against everybody else's belief about what his reality should be made a powerful impact on me — for him, hope was truly the inner strength that had been maintained in every stage of life.

## WHEN THE PROGNOSIS IS NOT SO GOOD . . .

The preceding paragraphs bear witness to the potentially powerful impact of hope on surviving a diagnosis of a life-threatening illness, but hope must be seen by carers and patients as something more than that which is invested only in prolonged mortality or immortality (Simsen, 1988:33). While it is undoubtedly perceived by some individuals with cancer as an important factor in their fight to maintain, regain, or augment health,

> hope does not necessarily have to focus exclusively on a cure or for more years of life (Hickey, 1986:134).

It can, in many ways, positively influence the quality of the life remaining, however little time may be left.

When the prognosis is not so good, hope may play a crucial role in promoting acceptance of illness-related limitations and dying (Hinds, 1988). For such patients, the focus has shifted from cure to coping more effectively with the inevitable. Owen (1989:76) suggests that when the cancer patient's focus shifts from hope of a cure to confronting issues that are not amenable to change

> coping effectively with losses due to the cancer process may depend on the individual's ability to maintain hope.

Another contribution to the discussion of the links between hope and effective coping is made by Herth (1989:67), who notes that philosophers, theologians, and writers have postulated hope as a phenomenon closely linked with a person's adaptive and coping powers.

Herth's study of the relationship between hope and coping enabled her to conclude that

when the patients' level of hope was high, level of coping was high (Herth, 1989:71).

The impact of hope on the ability of cancer patients to cope with their diagnosis and the limitations on their life was illustrated to me in a novel way during a social morning arranged for oncology and palliative care patients living in the community. These patients meet weekly with volunteers for recreational activities, general sharing of significant news and events, and a meal. A home-made hat was the chief prop for a crazy game of 'Who am I?' and amid much shouting and laughter, almost every rule of the game was broken. I cannot remember the last time I laughed so much in the company of a group of cancer patients. Several of them spoke of their determination to get the most out of the time left to them, including a woman attending for the first time. She was painfully thin, and I recognised in her the telltale signs often exhibited by people in the final phase of their illness. I took the opportunity for a quiet chat with her while we ate lunch, and was left full of admiration for the way in which she was coping with events that would surely have overwhelmed many people. She had adopted a policy of avoiding those who were negative in any way, as she believed this interfered with her single-minded focus on living to the full the life remaining. She had finally given up a range of outdoor activities, but was still able to turn out numerous handcrafted goods for the hospital's fund-raising activities. For this lady, indeed for all who attended that day, the life left was full of hope.

While it has been shown that some patients no longer expecting a cure use hope to enhance their general ability to cope with and adapt to the stresses associated with a terminal diagnosis, others focus their hopes more directly on specific and important aspects of life. This can range from the fairly broad objective of dying free from pain and with dignity with one's loved ones in attendance, to more specific, but tangible goals — the chance to bid farewell to a friend or relative not seen for many years; a final visit home to a long-nurtured garden; a last goodbye to a cherished pet; completion of a creative project; or an opportunity to be present at a significant family event, such as a wedding, christening, or birthday party.

This section has focused on the growing number of findings from cancer nursing research which suggest that people with cancer may remain positive and hopeful about the future in the face of the most hopeless situations. Elizabeth Kübler-Ross, renowned for her work with dying patients, suggests that all dying people maintain some hope, and can be nourished by it

even when confronted with knowledge of their impending death (cited by Yates, 1993:702).

# NURSING THE HOPE

The fact that nurses often assume a primary role in the care of patients with cancer places them in a strategic position to foster hope (Herth, 1990). This applies equally to patients undergoing active treatment and those for whom a cure may seem unlikely. Herth is not alone in her assumption that nurses must play a key role in the promotion of hope in people disgnosed with cancer. Chapman (1994) suggests that because nurses typically don't give out the hard facts, patients often turn to them for an injection of hope and assistance in confronting actual and potential losses during all phases of the cancer process. Owen (1989) sees a tendency to equate hope with the caring and compassionate nature of nursing as a reason for the expectation that nurses should play a key role in fostering or nurturing the development or preservation of hope. In apparent support of that expectation, Owen concludes that:

> Coping effectively with losses due to the cancer process may
> depend on the individual's ability to maintain hope. Hope, in
> turn, may help a person through adverse events, and its presence
> may precede positive coping. Nurturing hope, therefore, is
> offered as a nursing strategy designed to allay anxiety,
> depression, and fear in situations where the patient has no direct
> problem solving options (Owen, 1989:76)

An investigation by Rideout and Montemuro (1986) into the relationship between hope and morale, level of function and the physiological status of individuals with chronic heart failure found that patients who were more hopeful maintained their involvement in life, despite the physical limitations of their condition. These findings could be relevant to cancer patients, who experience limitations similar to those suffered by people with a range of chronic conditions. The authors concluded that the positive relationship between hope, morale, and level of function has implications for nursing practice, and that

> nursing, with its emphasis on caring, nurturing, and promotion of
> optimum health could deliberately enhance these characteristics
> in patients and promote adaptation (Rideout and Montemuro,
> 1986:430).

In order to facilitate promotion of hope in people with cancer, nurses often select strategies suggested by researchers examining the phenomenon of hope. Chapman (1994:56) devised a number of strategies from her work with breast cancer patients. These include empowerment of the patient by pointing out ways to gain control, encouraging the patient to discuss feelings openly, providing information about support groups for breast cancer patients and survivors, and suggesting therapeutic activities such as journal keeping, yoga, relaxation techniques, visual imagery, and art and music therapies. In a study exploring the meaning of hope, Herth (1990:1258) identified a range of hope-fostering and hope-hindering strategies which enabled her to develop a framework for nurses wishing to foster hope in terminally ill adults. Suggested strategies were quite diverse, ranging from sharing information on hope and dying, through encouraging closeness in order to foster a sense of belonging, actively listening and being present with the individual, and giving support and guidance when aims need to be refocused, to fostering lightheartedness through the appropriate use of humour and play. In a consideration of the role of the oncology nurse in enabling realistic hope, Hickey (1986:35–6) developed a range of nursing approaches towards this end. These were broadly categorised as

- developing an awareness of life,

- identifying a reason for living,

- establishing support systems,

- incorporating religion,

- incorporating humour, and

- setting realistic goals.

Like Herth, Hickey emphasised the importance of active listening as a key strategy. Poncar (1994:38) states that

> inspiring hope is an intervention that can be used with many nursing diagnoses, especially when feelings of helplessness, hopelessness, powerlessness, and depression are present.

Strategies for inspiring hope are concisely summarised by Poncar as incorporation of presence, touch, active listening, reality surveillance, and values clarification into encouragement offered by nurses to oncology patients.

Attempts to describe, understand, research, and conceptualise the experience of hope must remain an important and legitimate area of concern for nurses. Such attempts, facilitated by referral to the work of other nurse scholars, clinicians, and researchers, or by development of one's own studies, create for nurses an awareness of the variables that influence hope and coping. Without such awareness developing patient-centred strategies for facilitating adequate hope and effective coping will be difficult (Herth, 1989).

# HOPE AS A REALITY-BASED BELIEF . . . BUT WHOSE REALITY?

It would appear that there is some agreement about both the role of hope as an important coping strategy for cancer patients, and the key role played by nurses in promoting such hope. A range of diverse views put forward by clinicians and researchers in the field of cancer care indicates that the issue of realistic versus unrealistic hope is less clear cut. Raleigh

(1992) refers briefly to this issue, and appears to support a straightforward view that unrealistic hope is not beneficial to the healing process. Hickey (1986) considers the issue in more depth, and identifies 'realistic' hope as practical hope, then continues, with no hint of doubt, to label specific examples of hoping as realistic or nonrealistic. While acknowledging 'false' hope may be useful for a short time, as patient and family summon the reserves and coping skills needed to deal with the cancer experience, Hickey stresses that nurses should avoid encouraging false hope. Their role is to help patients to distinguish between realistic and false hope, while pushing them towards realistic hopefulness. In referring to the 'controversy' over the sanctioning of 'unrealistic' hope, Poncar (1994) assumes a similar position to Hickey. Hope may be promoted by the nurse if it is reality based, but should be modified, changed to a wish, or changed to a new hope if no longer grounded in reality.

Others see the debate surrounding this issue as far more problematic, including Yates (1993:703) who notes that:

> . . . there are no clear guidelines in the nursing literature as to whether there is a 'real' distinction between realistic and unrealistic hope, whether a certain level of hope or certain type of hope is detrimental, if hope is beneficial only if it is realistic and, if this is the case, just what realistic hope is.

Yates's review of the literature identifies the notion that people with a potentially terminal illness who demonstrate high levels of hope are in some way not accepting of reality. Underlying that notion is an assumption that there is a distinction between 'realistic' hope and 'unrealistic' hope in the context of dying. In response to this position Yates questions whether such an assumption refers to the reality of the health professional or the reality of the patient, and suggests that, as individuals construct their own reality on the basis of their own beliefs and experiences, the two realities are likely to be quite different (Yates, 1993:703).

Hall (1990:178) also devotes considerable attention to this debate, referring to Stoner's pinpointing of' 'two opposing theoretical views of hope and terminal illness'. The first view depicts hope as appropriate only if realistic. Hall's own discussions with nurses and other health care professionals reveal the prevalence of this view, as she invariably met with suggestions that she was 'encouraging denial' when presenting her ideas about hope in those diagnosed with cancer (Hall, 1990:179). Other examples of this view noted by Hall include McGee's claim that

> persons who experience unrealistically high levels of hope may be immobilised in the face of crisis (cited by Hall, 1990:179),

and a distinction between hoping, which is realistic, and 'wishing' which labels people's unrealistic wanting of things (Hinds, cited by Hall, 1990).

The second theoretical view identified by Stoner (cited by Hall, 1990:178) suggests that, as the purpose of hope is to

> maintain emotional well-being in the face of both ordinary and
> dire circumstances,

it has definite and positive value at all times. In supporting this view Hall presents the argument that everyone living is also dying, but, rather than dwelling on that fact, we are supposed to have hope for the future, however uncertain that might be. She continues this line of argument by suggesting that:

> . . . since the survival rates of the nondiagnosed are seldom
> predicted, it is clearly their prerogative to continue to live; they
> are not expected to prepare for death even though death may be
> just around the corner (Hall, 1990:179).

Why, questions Hall, should somebody receiving a medical diagnosis of cancer lose the right to remain hopeful? Why is it

> then and then alone that we say 'Now you are ill and you are
> dying. You must not continue to have hope in the same way as
> the rest of us do' (Hall, 1990:180)?

In dismissing this position, Hall suggests that the view that hope is inappropriate is the most defeating aspect of contact between those with advanced cancer and their nurses and physicians. In a final powerful statement, Hall accuses professional carers of lowering the quality of years left to the person when they see hope in the terminally ill and label it as denial. Who better to make such an accusation than a person still alive seven years after a diagnosis of metastatic cancer?

# CONCLUSION

Rather than presenting definite and clear-cut answers, this chapter set out to explore the premise that hope is a complex, multidimensional concept of considerable importance to people with potentially terminal conditions, including cancer. The fact that the chapter raises more questions than it answers suggests that continued questioning of the assumptions underlying this debate is a must for nurses and others associated with those suffering from cancer. Simsen (1988:38) supports and neatly summarises this position by stating that:

> To the hopeless person there is no way out. No other possibilities
> than those dreaded are seen, or sought. Left to himself (sic), the
> person unable to hope will build on to the circumstances of his
> (sic) imprisonment from the inside. For most people, the skill of
> hoping results in a fluctuating course between hopefulness and
> hopelessness. This is where the nurse has a vital part to play in
> supporting the hoping skill.

# References

Bolander VR (ed.) (1994): *Sorensen and Luckman's Basic Nursing: A Psychophysiologic Approach* (3rd edn). USA: W.B. Saunders Company.

Chapman K (1994): When the prognosis isn't as good. *RN* July: 55–57.

Fryback PB (1993): Health for people with a terminal diagnosis. *Nursing Science Quarterly* 6 3: 147–159.

Hall B (1990): The struggle of the diagnosed terminally ill person to maintain hope. *Nursing Science Quarterly* 3 4: 177–184.

Herth K (1989): The relationship between level of hope and level of coping response and other variables in patients with cancer. *Oncology Nursing Forum* 16 1: 67–72.

Herth K (1990): Fostering hope in terminally-ill people. *Journal of Advanced Nursing* 15: 1250–1259.

Hickey S (1986): Enabling hope. *Cancer Nursing* 9 3: 133–137

Hinds P (1988): Adolescent hopefulness in illness and health. *Advances in Nursing Science* 10 3: 79–88.

Nowotny M (1989): Assessment of hope in patients with cancer: Development of an instrument. *Oncology Nursing Forum* 16 1: 57–61.

O'Connor A, Wicher C, Germino B (1990): Understanding the cancer patient's search for meaning. *Cancer Nursing* 13 3: 167–165.

Owen D (1989): Nurses' perspectives on the meaning of hope in patients with cancer: A qualitative study. *Oncology Nursing Forum* 16 1: 75–79.

Poncar P (1994): Inspiring hope in the oncology patient. *Journal of Psychosocial Nursing* 32 1: 33–38.

Post-White J, Ceronsky C, Kreitzer MJ, Nickelson K, Drew D, Mackey KW, Koopmeiners L, Gutknacht S (1996): Hope, spirituality, sense of coherence, and quality of life in patients with cancer. *Oncology Nursing Forum* 23 10: 1571–1579.

Raleigh EDH (1992): Sources of hope in chronic illness. *Oncology Nursing Forum* 19 3: 443–448.

Rideout E, Montemuro M (1986): Hope, morale and adaptation in patients with chronic heart failure. *Journal of Advanced Nursing* 11: 429–438.

Rustoen T (1995): Hope and quality of life, two central issues for cancer patients: A theoretical analysis. *Cancer Nursing* 18 5: 355–361.

Simsen B (1988): Nursing the spirit. *Nursing Times* 84 37: 31–32.

Yates P (1993): Towards a reconceptualization of hope for patients with a diagnosis of cancer. *Journal of Advanced Nursing* 18 5: 701–706.

## Suggested reading

Dossey BM (1995): Peaceful Deathing and Death. In: Dossey BM, Keegan L, Guzetta KE, Kolkmeier LG (eds) *Holistic Nursing: A Handbook for Practice* (2nd edn). USA: Aspen.

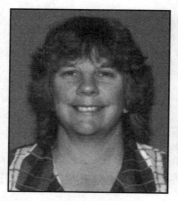
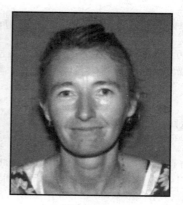

Stephanie Wellard

Trish Joyce

## STEPHANIE WELLARD
**Post Basic Chemotherapy Nursing Certificate; Graduate Diploma in Health Education, Lincoln Institute, Melbourne; Graduate Diploma in Health Administration, La Trobe University**
**Nurse Manager, Chemotherapy Unit, Peter MacCallum Cancer Institute**

Stephanie has been employed at the Peter MacCallum Cancer Institute for many years as a Clinical Nurse Consultant specialising in chemotherapy administration and education. Her major interests centre around patient education and the psychosocial aspects of patient care. Much of Stephanie's time is devoted to developing educational resources for both people with cancer and people who work with them.

Stephanie teaches in courses run by the Department of Nursing Education at Peter Mac, specialising in sexuality, cytotoxic administration and the ethical and legal aspects of chemotherapy nursing.

## TRISH JOYCE
**Graduate Diploma in Cancer Nursing, Registered Nurse**

Trish Joyce is a clinical nurse specialist in the haematology unit at Peter MacCallum Cancer Institute and a clinical nurse consultant in the Institute's day chemotherapy unit. She holds a Graduate Diploma in Cancer Nursing and is at present undertaking a Master of Health Science degree at the Victoria University of Technology.

# Chapter 6

## *Cancer and sexuality — a neglected issue?*

Cancer is an existential no-man's-land. As Aimee-Lee Ball suggested in the American magazine *Harper's Bazaar* (1995:339) it is a stage that is not quite life or death, but rather a nondescript continuum caught somewhere in between. In this no-man's-land there is no place for sexuality, only for the personal battle to survive.

This description is, of course, entirely wrong. The diagnosis of cancer threatens a person's wellbeing, but it may not curb their sexuality. If anything there is a greater need for intimacy at this time. As Hogan (1980) suggests, sexuality reflects everything about us — our true character —so it is more than just our sexual orientation. Stuart and Sundeen (1979) argue that sexuality is fundamental to the totality of the person and an integral factor in the uniqueness of every individual.

The World Health Organisation defines sexual health as

> the integration of the somatic, emotional, intellectual, and social aspects of a human being in ways that are positively enriching and will enhance personality, communication, and love (cited in Hughes, 1996).

Hughes contends that there are many ways of expressing sexuality, encompassing body image, perceptions of male and female roles, and interpersonal expressions of affection. Social and family roles and personal sexual preferences also impact upon this definition.

Such holistic definitions, however, are often ignored by the modern-day marketers' sexual titillations. As Weiss (cited in Shell, 1996:835) emphasised:

> Sexuality is [not] really about the things we've been taught to think it is . . . [It] isn't about intercourse or having babies . . . [It] isn't about

> competition and beauty contests or proving ourselves more beautiful
> or sexy than others . . . [It] isn't even only having orgasms and other
> pleasurable physical sensations. Sexuality is about connecting our
> head with our gut through our heart. It's about genuinely caring for
> ourselves, finding ecstasy in simply being alive, and giving voice to
> our ideas and feelings.

In other words, sexuality incorporates the physiological and psychological
aspects of being with interpersonal events, all of which interact to constitute
the person as a human being. Health carers should always be mindful of this.
If a person's sexuality is ignored, it could imperil their recovery, and leave
unaddressed issues that have the potential to cause personal distress (Metcalfe
and Fischman, 1985).

But health care workers still find it difficult to broach the subject of sexuality
with their patients. Perhaps the reticence stems from inherited cultural myths,
not to mention social inhibitions, which have clouded society's attitudes
towards sexuality. Maybe the most prevalent and damaging myth, which the
media dexterously manipulates, is that sexuality belongs to the young, the
beautiful and the able-bodied. If this is the case, those with disabilities or
disfigurements are excluded from this myth, as are those with cancer. How can
they possibly live up to the media mirage of the body beautiful image; and,
more importantly, what effect does the latter have on their quality of life?
Ferrans (1990) maintains that a person's quality of life is reflected in their sense
of wellbeing which, in turn, emanates from their satisfaction with the areas of
life that are important to them. Cancer and its treatment significantly alter
sexual expression, leading to a decreased sense of wellbeing and self-esteem,
and leaving the patient physically and psychologically incapable of meeting the
specified cultural aesthetic. Invariably, it adversely affects their quality of life.

## THE EFFECTS OF CANCER ON SEXUALITY

The diagnosis of cancer can dramatically alter a person's life. As one cancer
breast cancer survivor declared:

> Those old normals [in life] don't exist anymore, it's gone . . . Now
> what we have [are] new normals . . . You want it to go back to what
> it was like before . . . The cancer took my old life away (Pelusi,
> 1997:1345).

Not surprisingly, the psychological ramifications of a cancer diagnosis can have
a profound affect on a patient's sexuality. Without warning the patient is forced
to confront his/her mortality, in most cases for the first time. Survival issues
take priority over pre-existing concerns, often placing strains on personal
relationships. The patient may also be concerned about the reaction of friends
and family to their illness. Some patients feel an increased need to be touched
by their partner rather than to engage in sexual activity. The partner may
interpret this not as the patient's longing for reassurance, but as a slight to

them personally. The patient may also experience anger, frustration, depression, lowered self-esteem, guilt, fear of contamination and isolation; all of which adversely affect their sexuality.

The disease's physical symptoms also play their part. Fatigue, pain, anorexia and shortness of breath can reduce sexual desire and inhibit sexual expression. The direct effects of the cancer, such as erectile dysfunction related to neoplasms of the spinal cord, can be devastating. Physical disfigurements — particularly in the cases of head and neck cancers, cutaneous lymphomas and skin cancers — can negatively affect body image. Feelings of shame and embarrassment can affect intimacy, leading to sexual inhibition or abstinence. Even before the commencement of any cancer treatment the patient's sexual health has dramatically altered.

## THE EFFECTS OF TREATMENT ON SEXUAL HEALTH

Multi-modality treatments are now offered to cancer patients. These treatments include:

- surgery,
- chemotherapy,
- radiotherapy,
- biotherapy and
- endocrine manipulation.

One or a combination of these modalities may be used. Apart from their direct effects on sexual functioning, the health care worker must also be aware of systemic side effects. These may include nausea and vomiting, diarrhoea, alopecia, fatigue, pain, constipation, insomnia, mucositis, thrombocytopenia, immunosuppression and anaemia.

All of these can inhibit sexual expression and functioning, and, in particular, reduce the patient's libido. The role of health care workers is to offer the patient simple suggestions, so as to maximise the latter's comfort and wellbeing, thereby enabling them to remain sexually active. The patient should be encouraged to take analgesia prior to sexual activity in order to allay discomfort, or plan intercourse for times when they are most energetic. The importance of touch should be stressed for periods when sexual intercourse is contraindicated.

In addition, there are specific side effects. The patient's gonadal functioning will be disrupted. This can be a direct effect of the chemotherapy, radiotherapy or surgery and, in the case of chemotherapy and radiotherapy, can happen both during and after the treatment.

# The hypothalamic pituitary gonadal axis

Normally gonadal function is regulated by the hypothalamus and anterior
pituitary gland through a negative feedback system. The hypothalamus releases
the gonadotropin-releasing hormone which, in turn, stimulates the anterior
pituitary gland to release the follicle stimulating (FSH) and the lutenising (LH)
hormones. FSH regulates a woman's ovarian development and maturation,
while LH controls the development of ovulation and corpus luteum. The
ovaries produce oestrogen and progesterone, and, through a negative feedback
system with the hypothalamus and anterior pituitary gland, the secretion of FSH
and LH either increases or decreases depending on the stage of the ovarian
cycle. In men, FSH initiates, and is responsible for, the conversion of
spermatogonia into spermatocytes, while LH stimulates the cells of Leydig to
produce testosterone.

**Figure 6.1 The hypothalamic, pituitary, gonadal axis**

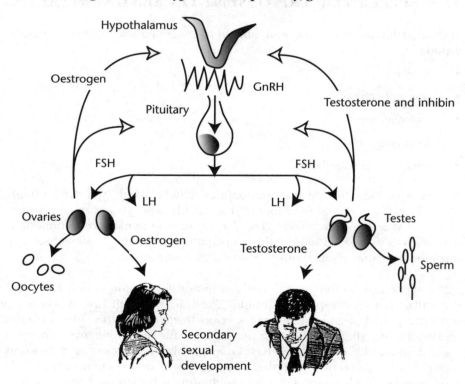

*The secretion of gonadotropin-releasing hormone from cells in the
hypothalamus controls the pulsatile release of LH and FSH from the pituitary
gland. These, in turn, regulate gamete production and sex steroid biosynthesis
at the gonadal level. Feedback of sex steroids occurs at the pituitary and
hypothalamic levels.*

(From Michael C. Perry (1996): The Chemotherapy Source Book, 2nd edn, published by Williams
& Wilkins. Used by permission of the copyright holder — Williams and Wilkins.)

The damage done to the ovarian follicles and germinal epithelium during and after chemotherapy and radiotherapy causes severe hormonal imbalances, resulting in the loss of the negative feedback system, and the elevation of FSH and LH levels, which are the hallmarks of primary gonadal failure. In women gonadal failure is initially characterised by irregular menstrual cycling which later progresses to amenorrhoea. However, during normal ovulatory cycles, it is still possible for the woman to conceive. Hormonal analysis will reveal increased levels of FSH and LH, and decreased levels of oestrogen and progesterone. In men, semen analysis will show oligospermia (a reduced number of sperm in the ejaculate) or azoospermermia (an absence of sperm in the ejaculate).

## Effects of chemotherapy on gonadal function

The effects of chemotherapy on sexual and reproductive function is determined by:

- the type of drug,
- the cumulative dose,
- the duration of the treatment,
- the patient's gender and age, and
- the length of time that has elapsed since the treatment (Groenwald et al., 1997; Klein, 1996; Shell, 1996).

The most notorious cause of infertility in both men and women are the alkylating agents, though other chemotherapeutic agents are also implicated (see Table 6.1).

### *Gonadal dysfunction in men*

Men are more susceptible to the effects of chemotherapy on gonadal function than women because of the high rate of mitotic activity associated with spermatogenesis. Oligospermia, azoospermia or permenant sterility can occur depending on the drug type, its dosage, and the patient's age. The time that has elapsed since the last treatment also will have a bearing on gonadal function and, if fertility is to return, it may do so within five to 49 months (Shell, 1996). Males experiencing puberty are more susceptible to gonadal injury than their prepubertal counterparts, who are afforded some protection because their germ cell development has not yet commenced. However, there is a drug threshold dose, and gonadal damage will occur if this is exceeded (Lamb, 1991).

Research into gonadal toxicity in males has focused predominantly on patients with Hodgkin's disease and testicular cancer. These patients are predominantly afflicted during their reproductive years, and, as their prognosis is excellent, long-term follow-up of this patient group provides valuable information. Oommen (1991) examined the effects of chemotherapy on 20 patients treated for Hodgkin's disease, all of whom achieved clinical remission.

**Table 6.1 Chemotherapeutic agents affecting sexual or reproductive function**

| Agent | Complication |
|---|---|
| *ALKYLATING AGENTS* | |
| Busulfan<br>Chlorambucil<br>Cyclophosphamide<br>Melphalan<br>Nitrogen mustard | Amenorrhoea, oligospermia, azoospermia, decreased libido, ovarian dysfunction, erectile dysfunction |
| *ANTIMETABOLITES* | |
| Cytosine arabinoside<br>5-fluorouacil<br>Methotrexate | As for alylating agents |
| *ANTITUMOUR ANTIBIOTICS* | |
| Doxorubicin<br>Plicamycin<br>Dactinomycin | As for alylating agents |
| *PLANT PRODUCTS* | |
| Vincristine | Retrograde ejaculation, erectile dysfunction |
| Vinblastine | Decreased libido, ovarian dysfunction, erectile dysfunction |
| *MISCELLANEOUS AGENTS* | |
| Procarbazine | As for alkylating agents |
| Androgens | Masculinisation (women) |
| Antiandrogens | Gynecomastia, impotence |
| Oestrogens | Gynecomastia, acne |
| Antioestrogens | Irregular menses |
| Progestins | Menstrual abnormalities, change in libido |
| Aminoglutethimide | |
| Corticosteroids | Masculinisation (women) |
| Interferons | Irregular menses, acne |
| pelvic pain | Transient impotence, amenorrhoea, |

(Reprinted, with permission of the publishers, from Groenwald SL, Goodman M, Hansen Frogge M, Henke Yarbro C (eds), *Cancer Nursing Principles and Practice*, 4th edn, published by Jones and Bartlett Publishers.)

The chemotherapy regimens used included MOPP (mustine hydrochloride, vincristine, procarbazine and prednisolone); COPP (cyclophosphamide, vincristine, procarbazine and prednisolene); and COP (cyclophosphamide, vincristine and prednisolone). Oommen found azoospermia and severe oligospermia in 93.7 per cent of the patients, while 86.5 per cent recorded high levels of circulating FSH and LH hormones, indicating gonadal damage. The recovery of spermatogenesis may take several years but this will be determined by the cumulative dose.

The gonadal toxicity associated with these regimens prompted a search for alternative regimens. Doxorubicin, bleomycin, vinblastine and dacarbazine (ABVD) is now the regimen of choice for advanced Hodgkin's disease because it is less likely to cause gonadal toxicity and is equally effective at inducing long-term remissions (Santora et al., 1987).

### Gonadal dysfunction in women

The effects of chemotherapy on the female's ovarian function are also related to the type of drugs used, their cumulative dosage, and the patient's age. Histological examinations of ovaries which had sustained cytotoxic damage revealed fibrosis and follicle destruction (Lamb, 1991). The destruction manifests in irregular menstrual cycles, amenorrhoea, elevated levels of FSH and LH, and decreased estradiol levels. The clinical symptoms of decreased estradiol levels include:

- vaginal epithelium,

- atrophy and dryness,

- hot flushes and

- dysparunia.

Age also plays a role. Because younger women have a larger complement of oocytes, they are less likely to develop permanent ovarian damage. Furthermore, women under the age of 30 are less likely than their older counterparts to develop permanent amenorrhoea. Nonetheless, younger women who are treated with chemotherapy may develop premature menopause. As with the male, a threshold drug dose does exist above which infertility will occur regardless of age. Prepubertal and pubertal girls appear to be less sensitive than their elders, though more research is required on the long-term effects on these patients (Klein, 1996).

### Menopause

Although cancer treatments are successfully prolonging life, women are often confronted with a premature menopause as a result of the treatment. As one cancer survivor declared:

> The instant menopause has drastically affected my sexuality. Cancer is gone, but life is not the same (Wilmoth and Ross, 1997:354).

The term menopause refers to the last menstrual period. It is a retrospective diagnosis. A woman is defined as post-menopausal when no periods have occurred for one year. However, women may be suffering from decreasing oestrogen levels for some years prior to this. These women are referred to as peri-menopausal or climacteric. Unlike the documentation of menopause in the healthy population, little research has been done into cancer survivors and how they experience this time in their lives, and very little literature exists to help women cope with the distressing symptoms of premature menopause. Dow (1995) suggests that moderate to severe menopausal symptoms are common amongst women treated with hormonal therapy or chemotherapy for endometrial, cervical and breast cancer and these are exceptionally problematic for younger women.

The signs and symptoms of menopause are related to changing levels of circulating oestrogens. The most commonly reported symptom, and that which is most discomforting for woman, are vasomotor disturbances. These include night sweats, hot flushes and palpitations, all of which cause undue stress and interruption to lifestyle. Because some of these symptoms may mimic the onset of cancer the fear that cancer may be returning can be a major source of anxiety for patients in remission. Other symptoms include:

- mood swings,

- depression,

- vaginal dryness,

- decreased libido and

- skin changes (Mayer and Linscott, 1995).

Also, as oestrogen production decreases, there is an increased incidence of cardiovascular disease and osteoporosis in the years following menopause (Wren, 1997).

But it is not only physical effects that need to be considered. Psychological effects of menopause can have a profound effect on a woman's sexuality. Women sometimes perceive menopause as a threat to womanhood and their role in life. For many, the menstrual cycle is essential to feminine identity. There are also cultural implications to be considered; for example Italian and Macedonian women view the onset of menopause as a sign of diminishing health. They consider the absence of their monthly flow of blood weakens their bodies and, as a result, their health suffers (Gifford, 1991). A premature menopause in these women can have profound effects.

Other women consider menopause as a sign of premature aging and feel they are been robbed of their youth. For many women Wilson's portrayal of the post-menopausal woman (as cited in Fenlon, 1995:168) lives on some 30 years later:

> After menopause the breasts begin to shrivel and sag. [The] breast becomes pendulous, wrinkled and flabby. The breasts lose their erotic sensitivity and sometimes do not respond to painful stimuli. Only timely oestrogen can prevent this premature decline of a woman's symbol of femininity.

***How can nurses assist women to adapt to the changes in their health during premature menopause?***

It is vital that nurses discuss with women before treatment commences the possibility of a premature menopause as a consequence of the treatment. This information and education will help prepare women for this period in their lives and reduce the stress and anxiety that affects nurses as a result of a poorly informed patient. Nurses often feel frustrated at the lack of information available to assist in the management of pre-menopausal symptoms in cancer patients.

A discussion about menopause should include the reason for menopause occurring and an explanation of the symptoms that may manifest themselves. Practical advice can assist women to manage some symptoms:

- Dress in comfortable clothing (cotton is better than synthetics).

- Eat a calcium-rich diet (between 1000 and 1500mg per day) that is low in fat and high in fibre.

- Reduce alcohol and caffeine intake.

- Use a water-based lubricant during sexual intercourse.

- Exercise regularly, particularly weight-bearing exercise.

- Learn and use relaxation strategies such as meditation, yoga etc.

- Join a support group — often discussion with other women going through menopause can be reassuring.

Moadel et al. (1995) studied psychosexual adjustment among women receiving hormone replacement therapy (HRT) for premature menopause following cancer treatment. They found that, compared with healthy women undergoing normal menopause, women receiving HRT for premature menopause experienced greater physical symptoms and psychological distress. The researchers concluded that HRT was necessary but not necessarily sufficient for the sexual rehabilitation of premature menopausal cancer survivors.

The HRT debate can be confusing and can give conflicting information to women experiencing early menopause. HRT has three major advantages associated with its long-term use:

1. Symptoms such as hot flushes, dry vagina, loss of libido and dysparunia will respond favourably to adequate oestrogen therapy.

2. It also helps prevent bone loss and reduces the risk of osteoporotic fractures.

3. It contributes to a reduction in heart disease and stroke. (MacLennan, 1991, suggests that heart disease and stroke are reduced by 50 per cent in users of HRT as compared with non-users.)

For the majority of women the risk of developing cancer is a major deterrent to taking HRT. There is no clinical data to support the rationale of withholding HRT in women with a previous gynaecological history of gestational trophoblastic disease, or of carcinoma of the vulva, cervix or ovary, with the possible exception of the endometrioid epithelial ovarian cancer (Smith et al., 1996). Similarly there is no evidence to suggest that HRT increases the risk of recurrence in non-gynaecological cancers such as lymphomas, leukemias and gastrointestinal cancers. The effects of HRT on breast cancer remains controversial. One of the main reasons for this controversy is the lack of prospective, randomised, placebo-controlled trials. Until guidelines are clearly established, recommendations regarding HRT in cancer survivors must be individualised.

## Fertility following blood cell/bone marrow transplantation

The use of high-dose treatment and blood cell/bone marrow transplantation in the treatment of haematological malignancies and some solid tumours has expanded rapidly over the last decade. More young people are now undergoing this treatment. However, there is still a dearth of knowledge concerning the impact of this treatment on reproductive function. Klein (1996) suggests that, while there have been many published reports of young women conceiving and giving birth to normal children, few studies detail women who wish to conceive in the future.

There have been a few reports of pregnancies and deliveries of normal children in women with aplastic anaemia treated with allogeneic bone marrow transplantation. However, the majority of these patients were young, had received no previous induction or consolidation chemotherapy and no total body irradiation as part of their conditioning regimen (Ostroff and Lesko, 1991). The addition of total body irradiation to the conditioning regimen is a major risk to fertility (Sanders, 1993).

More information in this area is required. Long-term follow-up regarding hormone levels and assessing the fertility status of both men and women are required if accurate information is to be provided regarding reproductive implications of high-dose ablative treatment.

## Effects of radiotherapy on sexual health

Radiotherapy plays a major role in the management of many cancers. Radiotherapy may be used in combination with other treatment modalities such as surgery, chemotherapy, hormone therapy and biotherapy in the cure, control and palliation of the disease. A person's sexuality may be affected by all treatment modalities and when radiation is given in combination it may be difficult to isolate the specific cause of the sexual dysfunction.

## Gonadal dysfunction due to radiotherapy

Radiation therapy may cause sexual and reproductive problems through primary ovarian failure in women and testicular aplasia in men, which may result in temporary or permanent sterility.

## Gonadal dysfunction in women

Temporary or permanent sterility is related to:

- the dose,

- the size and site of the field irradiated,

- the age and fertility status of the woman and

- the period of time the ovaries are exposed to radiation.

Ovarian irradiation of 2 to 10 Gy may result in ovarian failure and sterility in women depending on the age of the person at the time of treatment. Movement of the ovaries out of the field of radiation by oophoropexy, with appropriate shielding, may help to maintain fertility. Sitton (1997) suggests that pre-menopausal women over the age of 30 may experience menopausal symptoms due to scattered radiation even after oophropexy, but the scattered radiation may not be sufficient to cause menopausal symptoms in younger women. Masden and associates (1995), in a retrospective study, documented pregnancies in 36 women who had normal menstrual function when diagnosed with Hodgkin's disease and who received mantle and para-aortic irradiation of 40 to 44 Gy. Scatter radiation dose to the ovary was calculated to be 3.2 Gy. There were 38 pregnancies in 18 of the women. All children were normal. Premature menopause was experienced by one of the 36 women in this study.

In addition to sterility or transient infertility, other sexual dysfunctional problems may occur depending on the site and field being treated. For example, when the vagina is included in the radiation field, women report sexual dysfunction related to vaginal shortening and stenosis, and decrease in vaginal lubrication and sensation resulting in painful intercourse and less enjoyment of sexual activity. Seibel (1982:1196) acknowledged this and reported that:

> patients treated with radiation therapy for gynaecological cancer experienced decrease in sexual enjoyment and libido, decreased frequency of intercourse, decreased ability to achieve orgasm and [decreased] opportunity for intercourse

Acute side effects of pelvic and abdominal irradiation may impact on sexual function and sexual pleasure including symptoms such as

- fatigue,

- diarrhoea,

- nausea,

- irritating skin reactions,

- dysuria and

- urinary frequency.

### Gonadal dysfunction in men

Temporary or permanent azoospermia is related to:

- age,

- dose,

- tissue volume and

- exposure time.

Radiation therapy has been shown to affect spermatogenesis in men. Even with testicular shielding, doses as low as .15 Gy to the gonadal area can produce oligospermia lasting 12 to 18 months (Hubbard and Jenkins, 1983). The majority of men treated by external beam irradiation to the pelvic and abdominal area may experience permanent or temporary impotence, thought to be caused by fibrosis of the pelvic vasculature or radiation damage to the pelvic nerves. Problems with sexual dysfunction — such as inability to achieve an orgasm, inability to ejaculate and decreased sexual pleasure — are commonly cited (Maher, 1997:211).

## The effects of surgery on sexual health

Various types of surgery can lead to extremely damaging effects on an individual's sexuality by causing infertility or sexual dysfunction. Surgical procedures to the pelvic region that could result in damage include:

- radical prostatectomy,

- penectomy,

- orchidectomy,

- radical hysterectomy,

- pelvic examination and

- radical vulvectomy.

Indirect effects can result from surgery to the pelvic region or any surgery that interferes with vascular or nerve supply to that area. Some of these types of surgery can result in hormonal imbalances which affect sexual response and function.

The fashioning of a stoma in colorectal cancer, regardless of type, may have a profound effect on self-image and sexual identity because stomas create a physical change in body image and alter elimination patterns. Problems related to odour, inability to control motions, changing of ostomy bags and pouches, leakages and accidents may create a situation that will inhibit the resumption or the initiation of an intimate sexual relationship following surgery.

In addition to the initial surgery, many people wi
adjuvant chemotherapy and radiotherapy which w
problems previously mentioned.

# BODY IMAGE

## Psychological effects

The psychological trauma of being diagnosed with can            ....ve a
negative impact on a person's self-image. In much of today's world, movies,
television, newspapers and magazines place great emphasis
on health and physical beauty. In Australia, there is also a major
preoccupation with an outdoor lifestyle. Perceived inability to measure
up to these images can contribute to a negative image and diminished
personal identity for many people including those undergoing treatment
for cancer. It is possible that all these factors combined can result in
clinical depression and a subsequent loss of libido. Ferrell et al. (1995)
suggest that such depression often goes undiagnosed. Nurses should be
aware of this phenomena when interviewing their clients and should
recommend appropriate intervention and referral. Depression is often
compounded by other aspects of living with cancer such as financial
concerns and role changes within the family unit.

## Physical effects

Changes to physical appearance from the effects of cancer and its
treatments can have a significant effect on self-image and sexual
identity. Following a radical neck dissection and hemiglossectomy a
patient remarked, 'I can't even kiss anyone due to the shape of my
mouth' (Metcalfe and Fischman, 1985:23). The facial disfigurement and
functional impairment resulting from head and neck cancer and its
treatment can be particularly devastating because the effects of the
disease can be seen immediately and our most basic needs — such
as eating, drinking, talking and even breathing — can be altered
dramatically by the effects of reconstruction surgery, tracheostomies
and nasogastric feeding tubes.

In our society women's breasts symbolise motherhood, nurturing,
child rearing and the traditional women's role. The breasts are also
viewed as an essential body part for seduction and sexual pleasure.
(Schain, 1985:200) commented: 'We live in a mammocentric era where
breasts are glamorized, idealized, and sensationalized'. Women today
equate body image, the sense of attractiveness, and personal worth
with sexuality and gender identity. The prospect of breast surgery and
associated treatment creates fear and concern about future survival
and also raises anxiety related to alterations to body image, loss of
femininity and changes in personal relationships. Physical symptoms

pecia, weight loss and skin changes coupled with, in women, the symptoms of treatment-related abrupt menopause, e overwhelming. These physical and systemic effects place an ormous strain on self-image and sexual identity. This view is supported by Shell et al. (1996):

> For many people, the process of becoming ill may distort how they view their bodies and cast doubt on their sexual identity and response. This may result from physical changes in body size and shape, loss of control over bodily functions and/or feelings of being diseased and unclean.

# NURSING MANAGEMENT OF SEXUAL HEALTH

There are two major areas in which nurses can intervene to ease the impact of the negative effects of cancer and its treatment on sexual health — reproductive counselling and sexual assessment and education.

## Reproductive counselling

People with cancer are confronted with the fear that their illness and its treatment might affect their chances of having children, leaving them with feelings of inadequacy, particularly with regard to the manner in which they identify with their gender. Pre-treatment counselling sessions with the patient and the patient's partner are essential to ensure that they make an informed decision about choosing the correct option for their circumstance. The following questions should be asked in the counselling session:

- Will the treatment result in infertility?

- Will any infertility be temporary or permanent?

- What alternative options are there for reproduction (e.g. ovum and sperm banking)?

- When can the couple safely begin to plan a family?

- What are the most appropriate methods of contraception for the couple?

## Egg freezing

In Australia this procedure is offered only at the Royal Womens Hospital in Melbourne. It is an experimental program and at the time of writing no pregnancies had been achieved. However, it does offer a sense of hope to women facing potentially sterilising treatment. This hope empowers a woman to focus on the future with the possibility of having the opportunity to parent.

The program involves the freezing of mature or immature oocytes depending on the patient's circumstance. Mature eggs are collected following a period of ovarian stimulation which requires injections of fertility drugs to induce the growth of a number of follicles each of which contains an egg. Utilising a laporoscopic procedure the follicles are punctured and the eggs are collected and frozen. But for some women time is of the essence and the urgency of treatment means that the eggs must be collected without delay so there is no time for injections. In this situation existing follicles can be aspirated to collect the eggs and/or the ovary or a portion of the ovary can be removed. A general anaesthetic is required for this procedure. The material is then frozen and stored until requested by the woman. After thawing, immature eggs will have to be cultured and artificially ripened before fertilisation can take place.

## Sperm banking

Sperm banking should be discussed with all men prior to commencing treatment for their cancer. This service may offer the patient a last chance for reproductive potential. Sperm banks request several ejaculates with an interval of two or three days between each ejaculate to allow for the sperm concentration to return to peak levels. For a select number of patients, however, urgent treatment is a priority so it is possible to collect only one specimen.

A percentage of patients who present will already have severely diminished sperm counts before any treatment is commenced. The reason for this is still unclear. Sweet et al. (1996) suggested that 33 per cent of patients with Hodgkin's disease and 24 per cent of patients with testicular cancer have severely diminished sperm counts. To surmount this problem the intracytoplasmic injection has been developed. This allows a single sperm to be injected into an egg, allowing fertilisation to take place even with only a small volume of poor-quality sperm. This method has resulted in good pregnancy rates when combined with the in vitro fertilisation. Men who cannot deliver several specimens can be assured that their potential to father children in the future can still be an option for them.

## Pregnancy and cancer

Breast cancer is the most common cancer in pregnant and post-partum women, occurring in 1:3000 pregnancies. Many women are now delaying their pregnancies so it is likely that this ratio will increase. Other malignancies most commonly associated with pregnancy are those seen during the child-bearing years:

- leukemia,

- lymphoma and

- malignant melanoma.

Caring for an expectant mother with cancer can be a very traumatising and emotional time for all concerned. In making the decision to treat the woman, a number of factors have to be taken into account, the most important of which is the gestation age of the foetus. Due to the teratogenic effects of the chemotherapy and radiotherapy, if possible, treatment should be postponed until after delivery. If immediate treatment is indicated it should be given only after the first trimester. Treatment after this period is generally not associated with a high risk of foetal malformation but may be associated with premature labour and foetal wastage. Klein (1996:826) suggests that the risks of teratogenic effects are highest in the first trimester,

> but even in this situation the recommendation for therapeutic abortion is controversial and often unnecessary.

Other factors affecting the decision to treat the expectant mother include:

- the health of mother and foetus at time of diagnosis;

- the prognosis of the mother and the likelihood of future pregnancies; and

- the known teratogenic effects of the drugs used and the dose (Shell, 1996).

Mutagenecity is another concern for patients who are considering parenthood after treatment. Mutagenesis refers to the genetic alterations expressed in future generations. Studies done in this area suggest that there is no detectable increase in congenital anomalies and chromosomal abnormalities in the offspring of cancer patients, and this appears to be consistent with the general population (Li et al., 1979; Senturia and Peckham, 1990; Mulvihill et al., 1987). However this area remains controversial and if accurate information is to be provided to future parents more scientific data is required.

## Family planning

People with cancer should be counselled not to start a family during their treatment to avoid the teratogenic and mutagenic effects of the treatment. A waiting time of two years from completion of treatment is recommended before a pregnancy should be planned. This allows for recurrence of disease to manifest and also allows for the recovery of ovarian function and spermatogenesis (Petrek, 1994). During counselling contraceptive methods should be discussed. A method should be chosen which is both safe and appropriate for that person. It is often difficult to predict when an individual receiving chemotherapy or radiotherapy is infertile therefore it is vital that the person continues to use contraception for some time after the cancer treatment has been completed until it has been clearly defined the patient has become infertile.

The greatest fear for the mother is that her cancer will be reactivated with the onset of pregnancy. According to Groenwald et al. (1997) pregnancy following cancer treatment has been extensively evaluated in breast cancer. Particularly with this malignancy there could be a potential for disease recurrence because of the hormonal changes that occur during pregnancy. Dansforth (1991) suggested that pregnancy does not appear to compromise the survival of women with a history of breast cancer. Decisions for and against pregnancy must be balanced against quality of life issues for that person. Decisions need to be made on an individual basis.

## Sexual assessment and education

Nurses play a pivotol role in assisting the patient with cancer to remain sexually active and feeling positive about their bodies during and following treatment. However, nurses and physicians remain reticent about openly discussing sexuality-related issues with their patients. Young-McCaughan (1996) described sexual functioning in women with breast cancer treated with adjuvant therapy. The majority of women in this study had not been asked by their doctor or nurse about sexual functioning issues. Similarly Wilmoth and Ross (1997) documented that women suffering sexual dysfunction from cancer treatment felt frustrated that health care professionals were not addressing their needs. Wilson and Williams (1988) surveyed 937 nurses. Of these 91 per cent agreed that discussing a patient's sexuality should be a routine component of nursing yet only 51 per cent reported that they were comfortable initiating this discussion. Many of these nurses wrote comments which indicated that their reluctance to discuss sexuality issues with their patients was based on a lack of knowledge. Merrill and Thornby (1990) put forward three main reasons why nurses fail to take a sexual history:

1.  embarrassment,

2.  failure to acknowledge that a sexual history is relevant to the presenting problem and

3.  feeling inadequately trained.

Nurses need to be aware of their own sexual attitudes, values and beliefs. This self-knowledge will assist them to respect other people's positions and discuss sexuality in a nonjudgmental manner.

### Homosexuality

> It must never be assumed that all patients have or wish to have a
> partner or that all partners are of the opposite sex (Shell, 1996:852).

If a patient does not appear to have a sexual partner it should not be assumed that they will not be affected by the sexual implications of cancer and its therapy. Homosexuals or single people do not come with a tag attached. When nurses are counselling patients, they must ensure that they do not make assumptions and personal judgements surrounding the sexual orientation of the person with cancer. With the increase in HIV-related cancers — in Australia approximately 4 per cent of new AIDS diagnoses are accounted for by non-Hodgkin's lymphoma (Chipman, 1997) — and with

AIDS in Australia being contained to the predominantly male homosexual population (Carr, 1992), it is more likely in the future than in the past that nurses will be counselling and educating homosexuals.

A homosexual relationship will experience much the same stress and strain as a heterosexual relationship. Discussions about the possibilities of treatment related to sexual dysfunction should take place with the patient and his/her partner. Shell (1996:412) acknowledged this and claimed that

> timely discussion of possible or probable sexual dysfunction and ways to manage it can help all couples tolerate treatment with less stress. Also the confidence that sexual problems have been recognized, or are being dealt with, and may be satisfactorily overcome, could inspire greater compliance with therapy.

It is not the nurse's role, however, to dwell on the sexual preferences of the patient; rather it is the responsibility of the nurse to offer advice on sexual health issues such as:

- fertility and contraception,

- treatment-related sexual dysfunction and

- safe sexual practice during and after treatment.

Advice can range from the use of lubricating creams to prevent friction-induced bruising and bleeding due to thrombocytopenia to advice on barrier contraception to reduce infection rates in people with neutropaenia and/or contamination from sperm containing possible cytotoxic metabolites.

## Discussing sex

Oncology nurses need to have an in-depth knowledge on how cancer and its treatment can affect sexual health. Cartwright-Alcarese (1995) stresses the importance of gaining a sexual history at the beginning of the treatment. This emphasises to the patient that it is a legitimate aspect of health care and that it is appropriate to discuss such concerns. It is important when discussing sexuality that the patient's privacy and confidentiality are assured.

A refusal to discuss such issues should be respected but does not mean that they should not be raised at a later time. Introducing the subject will open the door for the patient to raise questions in the future. The nurse does not have to be a sex therapist to assist these patients. However, whilst many sexual problems require only minimal intervention, complex problems can occur that require more expertise. In this situation, the nurse should refer the patient and his/her partner to a sex-therapist/counsellor.

The Annon model, commonly called the PLISSIT model, may be easily adapted and used for sexual counselling or as a nursing assessment tool. This model incorporates four levels of sexual counselling (see Table 6.2). Nurses may find that this model of counselling provides a useful framework for identifying pre-existing sexual health problems and to highlight sexual dysfunction and fertility concerns that may occur as a result of the cancer and its treatment.

---

### *Table 6.2 Annon model of approaches to sexual concerns*

**Permission:** Providing reassurance that the client is normal and has professional permission to continue what he or she has been doing. It is important that permission not be given for activities that are potentially harmful to the individual.

**Limited Information:** Providing information directly relevant to the client's concern. This can effect significant changes in the client's attitudes and behaviour.

**Specific Suggestions:** Direct efforts to assist the client to change behaviour in order to attain stated goals by providing specific suggestions directly related to the particular problem.

**Intensive Therapy:** Highly individualised therapy which is used when brief therapy is not effective.

---

(Adapted from Annon J: Behavioral Treatment of Sexual Problems: Brief Therapy: Vol 1, New York, Harper and Row, 1976. Reprinted from Fogel CI and Lauver D (1990): *Sexual Health Promotion*, by permission of the publishers, W.B. Saunders Company.)

### *Permission*

The first level of intervention introduces the topic of sexuality and allows the person or couple to identify any concerns they may have related to their present sexual practice and relationships. It would be appropriate at this time to discuss the effect that the cancer and treatment may have on sexual function and fertility.

### *Limited information*

The second level is the educational component in which the nurse provides specific information related to side effects of treatment and discusses the implications for sexual functioning and fertility. At this time it is useful to provide relevant educational literature, such as pamphlets or booklets focusing on the short-term and the long-term side effects of the appropriate treatment modality. People from non-English-speaking backgrounds should be provided with educational material in their own language.

### *Specific suggestions*

At the third level the nurse may respond to previously identified problems by giving detailed information, and suggesting strategies to help manage sexual health problems.

### Intensive therapy

The fourth level reveals the need for referral to a professional therapist if the sexual dysfunction problem is too complex or outside the nurse's level of expertise.

Nurses are well able to intervene at the first three levels, for example,

- taking a brief sexual history,
- inquiring about lifestyle and relationships, and
- providing information related to disease- or therapy-related side effects on sexual functioning.

In addition, giving specific suggestions that may alleviate the problem or improve sexual health are well within the oncology nurse's professional capabilities. Occasionally intensive sexual therapy or medical intervention is required and the nurse will need to recommend referral to a sex therapist or some other appropriate source.

# CONCLUSION

Nurses and other health professionals deal with sexual health issues frequently as part of their professional practice. The extent of their role in sexual health counselling, however, will depend on their level of expertise and their qualifications. To neglect this important area of cancer nursing is to not treat the person with cancer as a whole person. As early as 400 BC Plato remarked that the great error of his day in the treatment of the human person was the separation of the soul from the body (as cited in Renshaw, 1994:354). Nursing practitioners should always be mindful of the age-old wisdom.

## References

Ball AL (1995): Women are surviving cancer — breast, ovarian and uterine — in record numbers. The question is, how can they bring their sex lives out of remission? *Harper's Bazaar* March: 339–341.

Carr A (1992): What Is AIDS? In: Timewell E, Minichiello V, Plumber D (eds): *AIDS in Australia*. New York: Prentice Hall, p. 14.

Cartwright-Alcarese F (1995): Addressing sexual dysfunction following radiation therapy for a gynecological malignancy. *Oncology Nursing Forum* 22 8: 1227–1231.

Chipman MP (1997): HIV-related lymphoma. *Amgenda* 11: 11.

Dansforth D (1991): How subsequent pregnancy affects outcome in women with a prior breast cancer. *Oncology* 5: 23–30.

Dow KH (1995): A review of late effects of cancer in women. *Seminars in Oncology Nursing* 11 2: 128–136.

Fenlon D (1995): Menopause: A problem for breast cancer patients. *European Journal of Cancer Care* 4 4: 166–172.

Ferrans C (1990): Development of a quality of life index for patients with cancer. *Oncology Nursing Forum* 17: 15–21.

Ferrell BR, Dow KH, Leigh S, Ly J, Gulasekaran P (1995): Quality of life in long term cancer survivors. *Oncology Nursing Forum* 22 6: 915–922.

Gifford S (1991): Culture and breast cancer: Myth or mosaic? Unpublished paper submitted to the Department of Social and Preventative Medicine, Monash University, Melbourne.

Groenwald SL, Goodman M, Hansen Frogge M, Henke Yarbro C (1997): *Cancer Nursing Principles and Practice* (4th edn). Sudbury, Massachusetts: Jones and Bartlett Publishers.

Hogan R (1980): *Human Sexuality. A Nursing Perspective*. New York: Appleton-Century-Crofts.

Hubbard SM, Jenkins J (1983): An overview of current concepts in the management of patients with testicular tumours of germ cell origin — Part II: Treatment strategies by histology and stage. *Cancer Nursing* 6 2, April: 125–139.

Hughes MK (1996): Sexuality issues: Keeping your cool. *Oncology Nursing Forum* 23 10:1507–1511.

Klein CE (1996): Gonadal Complications and Teratogenicity of Cancer Therapy. In: Perry MC (ed.) *The Chemotherapy Source Book* (2nd edn). Baltimore: Williams & Wilkins

Krebs LU (1997): Sexual and Reproductive Dysfunction In: Groenwald SL, Hansen Frogge M, Goodman M, Henke Yarbro C: *Cancer Nursing Principles and Practice* (4th edn). Boston: Jones & Bartlett.

Lamb MA (1991): Effects of chemotherapy on fertility in longterm survivors. *Dimensions in Oncology Nursing* 5 4: 13–16.

Lamb MA (1990): Psychosexual issues: The woman with gynecological cancer. *Seminars in Oncology Nursing* 6: 237–243.

Li FP, Fine W, Jaffe N (1979): Offsrping of patients treated for cancer in childhood. *Journal of the National Cancer Institute* 62: 1193–1197.

MacLennan AH (1991): Hormone replacement therapy and the menopause. *Medical Journal of Australia* 155: 44–45.

Maher KE (1997): Male Genitourinary Cancers. In: Dow KH, Dunn BJ, Iwamoto R, Fieler V, Hinderley L, *Nursing Care in Radiation Oncology*. Philadelphia: W.B. Saunders.

Marsden BL, Gludice L, Donaldson SS (1995): Radiation induced premature menopause: A misconception. *International Journal of Radiation Oncology, Biology, Physics* 32: 1461–1464.

Mayer DK, Linscott E (1995): Information for women: Management of menopausal symptoms. *Oncology Nursing Forum* 22 10: 1567–1570.

Merrill JM, Thornby JI (1990): Why doctors have difficulties with sexual histories. *Southern Medical Journal* 83 6: 613–617.

Metcalfe MC, Fischman SH (1985): Factors affecting the sexuality of patients with head and neck cancer. *Oncology Nursing Forum* 12 2: 21–25.

Moadel AB, Ostroff JS, Lesko LM, Bajorunas DR (1995): Psychosexual adjustment among women receiving hormone replacement therapy for premature menopause following cancer treatment. *Psycho-Oncology* 4: 273–282.

Mulvihill JJ, McKeen EA, Rosner F, Zarrabi MH (1987): Pregnancy outcome in cancer patients. *Cancer* 60: 1143–1150.

Oommen R, Jose CC, Vishwanathan F, Roul SK, Singh AD (1991): Ovarian and testicular damage by cytotoxic drugs. *Indian Journal of Cancer* 28: 119–123.

Ostroff JS, Lesko LM (1991): Psychosexual Adjustment and Fertility Issues. In: Whedon MB (ed.): *Bone Marrow Transplantation. Principles, Practice and Nursing Insights*. Boston: Jones & Bartlett, pp. 312–333.

Pelusi J (1997): The lived experience of surviving breast cancer. *Oncology Nursing Forum* 24 8: 1343–1353.

Petrek JA (1994): Pregnancy safety after breast cancer. *Cancer* 74: 528–531.

Poorman SG (1988): *Human sexuality and nursing process*. Norwalk: Appleton & Lange.

Renshaw DC (1994): Beacons, breasts, symbols, sex and cancer. *Theoretical Medicine* 15: 349–360.

Sanders JE (1993): Growth and Development after Bone Marrow Transplantation. In: Forman SJ, Blume KE, Thomas ED (eds) *Bone Marrow Transplantation*. Boston: Blackwell Scientific Publications, pp. 527–537.

Santoro A, Bonadonna G, Valagussa P (1987): Longterm results of combined chemotherapy–radiotherapy approach to Hodgkin's disease: Superiority of ABVD plus radiotherapy versus MOPP plus radiotherapy. *Journal of Clinical Oncology* 5: 27–37.

Schain WS (1985): Breast cancer surgeries and psychosexual sequel: Implications for remediation. *Seminars in Oncology Nursing* pp. 200–205.

Seibel M, Freeman MG, Graves WL (1982): Sexual function after surgical and radiation therapy for cervical carcinoma. *Southern Medical Journal* 75 10: 1195–1197.

Senturia YD, Peckham CS (1990): Children fathered by men treated with chemotherapy for testicular cancer. *European Journal of Cancer* 26: 429–432.

Shell JA (1996): Impact of Cancer on Sexuality. In: Otto S (ed.) *Oncology Nursing* (3rd edn). St Louis: Mosby, pp. 835–858.

Shell JA (1991): *Knowledge Deficit Related to Radiation Therapy: Guidelines for Oncology Nursing Practice* (2nd edn). Philadelphia: W.B. Saunders, pp. 62–69.

Shell JA, Doherty ML, Bell KE (1996) Gonadal Toxicities. In: Liebman MC, Camp-Sorell D (eds), *Multimodal Therapy in Oncology Nursing*. St Louis: Mosby.

Sitton E (1997): Hodgkin's Disease and Non-Hodgkin's Lymphoma. In: Dow KH, Dunn BJ, Iwamoto R, Fieler V, Hinderley L, *Nursing Care in Radiation Oncology*. Philadelphia: W.B. Saunders.

Smith HO, Kammerer-Doak DN, Barbo BM, Sarbo GE (1996): Hormone replacement therapy in the menopause: A pro opinion. *A Cancer Journal for Clinicians* 46: 343–363.
Stuart GW, Sundeen SJ (eds) (1979): *Principles and Practice of Psychiatric Nursing*. St Louis: CV Mosby.

Sweet V, Servy EJ, Karrow AM (1996): Reproductive issues for men with cancer: Technology and nursing management. *Oncology Nursing Forum* 23 1: 51–58.

Wilmoth MAC, Ross JA (1997): Women's perception. Breast cancer treatment and sexuality. *Cancer Practice* 5 6: 353–359.

Wilson ME, Williams HA (1988): Oncology nurses' attitudes and behaviours related to sexuality of patients with cancer. *Oncology Nurses Forum* 15: 49–53.

Wren B (1997): Hormone replacement therapy. *Current Therapeutics* February: 14–23.

Young-McCaughan S (1996): Sexual functioning in women with breast cancer after treatment with adjuvant therapy. *Cancer Nursing* 19 4: 308–319.

*The discomfort associated with constipation has added to the bone and oral pain. This increase in discomfort means Mary has fewer reserves to cope with the nausea experienced. Her nutritional intake is small. Her sleep is disturbed through the pain and nausea.*

*Mary and her family are anxious about her worsening prognosis. She and her husband are also worried about the increase in morphine dose, and think she may become dependant on the drug. In addition, Mary is having problems juggling hospital appointments for her chemotherapy with her family responsibilities.*

Is this situation out of the ordinary? No, it is not unusual, and it illustrates well the complexities of cancer care. But while some situations may be difficult, patient management is always both challenging and satisfying.

# FACTS AND FALLACIES ABOUT CANCER PAIN

In many ways cancer pain is similar to other pain of a chronic nature. Differences lie in the unique connotations cancer has for those diagnosed and for those in a caring role.

The myths surrounding cancers and cancer pain are many and varied. These images are often negative:

- death and pain are linked to all cancer diagnoses (and usually in that order!);

- people with cancer all die in pain; and

- cancer pain cannot be controlled the way other pain can.

Erroneous images are a source of anxiety and a negative influence on therapeutic behaviour. Education is essential in helping to dispel these myths.

Some of the facts about cancer pain can also produce negative images. Whilst not all cancers cause pain, many do. Those people who have pain associated with cancer have been shown to complain of two to four separate pains (Cleeland et al., 1994; O'Connor, 1997). Pain is likely to increase with advancing disease, especially in the last 48 hours of life. Emotional distress related to diagnosis, prognosis and symptomatology contribute to the total suffering experienced.

Well-planned patient care is essential in minimising the negative impact of pain on the person with cancer and on the carers.

# DEFINITIONS OF PAIN

This chapter is introducing a broad concept of pain. Definitions focusing only on physical aspects do not adequately describe cancer pain. A definition must represent all facets of pain, including the physical, emotional, and psychosocial aspects.

Margo McCaffery, a North American nurse, has written extensively on the subject of pain. Her definition, outlined in the 1960s, has been widely accepted by nurses:

> Pain is whatever the experiencing person says it is, existing whenever the experiencing person says it does (McCaffery and Beebe, 1989:7).

The International Association for the Study of Pain (1979:250) defines pain as

> an unpleasant sensory and emotional experience, associated with actual or potential tissue damage, or described in terms of such damage.

A similar definition has been put forward by two oncologists:

> a subjective phenomenon that is unique to each individual . . . A chronic pain syndrome is an ongoing unpleasant sensation that may or may not be directly related to tissue damage, does not signal sudden physical change in bodily function, and often affects the [person's] behaviour and lifestyle (Casciato and Lowitz, 1988:50).

These definitions refer to the wider implications of pain. Pain in this context can be seen as 'suffering', and has been defined as such by various authors (Woodruff, 1996, Twycross, 1994). (See Figure 7.1.) It can be seen that the physical sensation of pain is only one slice in the overall pie of suffering.

**Figure 7.1 The concept of suffering**

Pain
+ physical symptoms
+ psychological problems
+ social difficulties
+ cultural factors
+ spiritual concerns
_____
= Total suffering

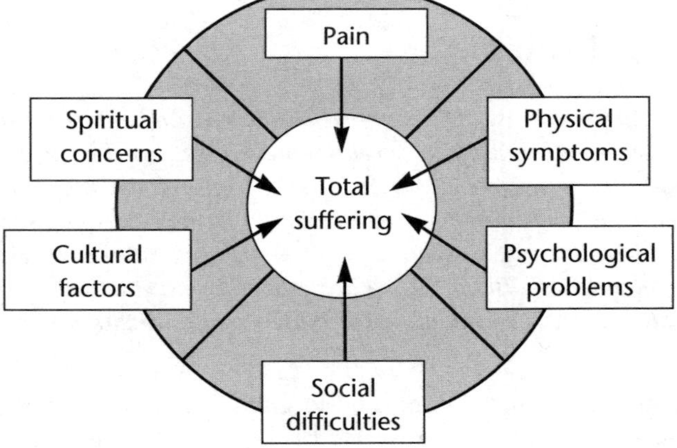

(Reproduced with permission from Woodruff R: *Palliative Medicine — Symptomatic and Supportive Care for Patients with Advanced Cancer and AIDS*, 2nd edition, 1996, Asperula, Melbourne)

Most definitions provide some information to fill in the complex picture of cancer pain. It must be remembered that pain is a psychological state, and a symptom that can be defined only by the person who has the pain, no-one else can experience that pain.

# THE SUBJECTIVE NATURE OF PAIN

McCaffery's definition focuses on the subjective nature of pain. This can present problems for health professionals trained in the collection of objective data to support hypotheses regarding patient problems. How, then, is a symptom that may have no observable component dealt with? In an attempt to 'prove' pain, information available is often filtered through the nurse's internal screens of validity. Is it reasonable for this person to be complaining of pain, and is the severity of pain to be expected?

As patient advocates, nurses must accept patients' reports about the presence and severity of pain as valid, the only valid measure for pain. The most important and difficult aspect of helping the person with pain is to accept and appreciate this fact. Subjective symptoms such as sadness and anxiety are accepted, and pain must be treated in the same way.

## Case history 2

*John Carr has undergone surgery for a perforated appendix. Post-operative orders include the administration of intramuscular pethidine 100mg every four hours as required. John is requesting his injection after three and a half hours.*

*Changes in vital signs are noted when John is in pain. Pulse and blood pressure increase, respirations become shallower, and his skin is pale and clammy. In addition, John verbalises both his pain and the effects of analgesia.*

## Case history 3

*Brian Brown is a 67-year-old single man with a primary adenocarcinoma of the rectum with liver and cerebral metastases, and is receiving a course of radiotherapy. Analgesia ordered is slow-release morphine, 180mg twice a day, with an 'as required' dose of 30mg (immediate-release solution) for break-through pain. He requires some assistance with activities of daily living due to his unsteadiness. Brian has a fair appetite, exhibits no change in vital signs or external appearance, and yet often complains of severe abdominal pain.*

It might feel more comfortable giving three to four hourly analgesia to John. He has an obvious cause for his pain, and signs can be observed to validate this. Brian, on the other hand, does not appear to be in pain. There may also be concerns in relation to overdosing, as he is already receiving 360mg of morphine per day.

# MISCONCEPTIONS ABOUT ANALGESIC PAIN CONTROL

Misconceptions about analgesic (and particularly morphine) use contribute to the problem of uncontrolled cancer pain (Foley, 1989; Rimer et al., 1987). Would someone pretend pain to secure analgesia? Can morphine overdosing occur? The answer to these questions is usually no.

Table 7.1 presents examples of misconceptions about analgesics often expressed by patients, their relatives and carers, and the corresponding accurate statement.

**Table 7.1 Facts and fallacies about pain control**

| MISCONCEPTION | FACT |
|---|---|
| • Morphine is addictive. | • Morphine does not lead to the development of psychological dependence (addiction) when used for the purposes of pain control.<br>• Physical dependence is an expected response and does not imply that morphine should not be used. |
| • Analgesics will lose their effects if used in early stages of disease. | • In the majority of cases, there is no upper limit, or 'ceiling dose' for morphine.<br>• The dose of analgesia required is the amount which reduces/relieves the pain to a level acceptable to the person experiencing pain. |
| • The side effects of analgesics can cause more distress than pain. | • Management of side effects should commence at the same time as initiation of analgesic therapy.<br>• Many side effects are temporary, and do not present long-term problems. |
| • Taking tablets regularly is not good for health. | • Regular analgesic dosing is an essential part of chronic pain management. |
| • Increasing the morphine dose in end-stage disease will cause respiratory depression and early death. | • Tolerance develops to most of the side effects of morphine, including the respiratory depressant effect. |

It is essential to challenge erroneous views and attempt to replace inaccurate knowledge with accurate information.

## Case history I continued

*Mary now has end-stage disease. Death is near, and her husband and son have been called. There is an order for morphine, 30mg subcutaneously as required, and Mary has been having this approximately hourly. She is becoming increasingly restless, disturbing the bedclothes, and occasionally groaning. Her husband and son are obviously distressed. Respirations are uneven and shallow, with a rate of 12–14 per minute. It is 40 minutes since Mary's last morphine dose.*

How do you feel about giving Mary her next dose? In light of the previous discussion, it can be seen that the most appropriate action is aimed at enhancing patient comfort, regardless of the dose requirements to achieve this aim.

## APPROACHES TO THE CLASSIFICATION OF CANCER PAIN

Exploring the physical characteristics and pathological changes associated with cancer pain provides practical information which can be used to plan effective interventions for pain management. In this way classifications provide a framework on which to build theoretically based clinical practice.

It is not the purpose of this chapter to explain the physiology of pain in great depth, but further reading is recommended. There are many excellent books and journals on this subject including those mentioned in the reference list at the end of the chapter.

A simplistic and widely used classification categorises cancer pain according to its intensity, using ratings of mild, moderate, and severe (World Health Organisation (WHO), 1986). Interventions are then chosen on the basis of pain severity.

**Figure 7.2 The WHO 3-step analgesic ladder for cancer pain**

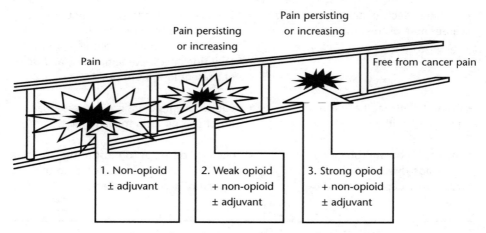

(Reprinted from *Pain Relief in Advanced Cancer* by Robert Twycross by permission of the publisher Churchill Livingstone)

Another classification looks at specific structures that can be involved in the malignant process. In this model the pain stimulus is defined as having a peripheral, central or psychogenic origin. Peripheral pains are further classified as involving superficial, intermediate or deep body structures, with the differentiating characteristics of each type outlined. Figure 7.3 presents such a classification that the author has found useful in conceptualising cancer pains.

***Figure 7.3 Analgesic ladder for cancer pain management based on diagnosis of origin of the pain***

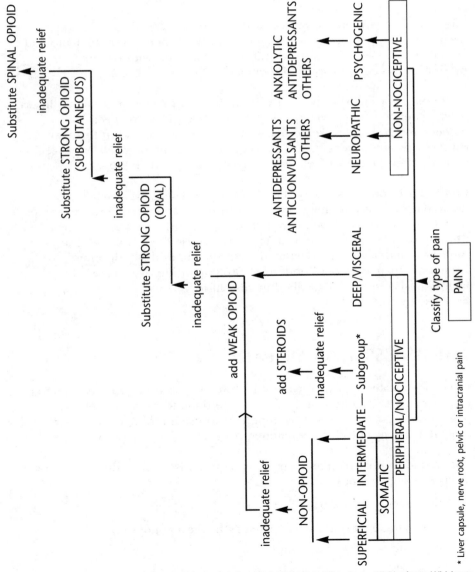

(Reprinted by permission of NM Muirden, KA Jackson, JM Bingham, WJ Moon: Pain Control/Palliative Care Unit, Peter MacCallum Cancer Institute)

Using this model, the rationale behind various pain management strategies becomes clear and the role of differing drugs is explained. It becomes easier to predict the type of pain a patient may experience, and ensure that preventive pain management strategies are in place.

It can be seen why the accurate assessment of pain is crucial to planning individualised pain management.

## ACUTE AND CHRONIC PAIN

The causes of pain in the person with cancer are varied. In addition to disease-related pain, cancer treatments can be a source of both acute and chronic pain. This is a useful classification for pain, with patient presentations and principles of treatment different for both.

Acute pain is usually associated with an injurious event or an acute illness. It has a defined cause which is usually physical. It often acts as a defence mechanism, warning that something is amiss, and in this way can be a positive event. Acute pains are of the duration of days or weeks, and are often linked to feelings of anxiety (Woodruff, 1996).

Chronic pain presents a very different picture. There may be actual tissue damage, or pain may occur as a result of abnormal body responses to past injury. There is often an increase in intensity of pain over time. Chronic pain lacks positive meaning, and is described as more of a 'situation' than an 'event'. Depression accompanies this pain more commonly than anxiety (Woodruff, 1996). Other life events are compromised, such as described in case history 1, with a resulting decrease in quality of life.

## THE ASSESSMENT OF PAIN

It has been stated that pain cannot be 'proved', so how can this symptom be measured in a reliable manner, as must be done to assess the efficacy of pain control interventions? It is important to use a tool that can describe pain accurately, in a reproducible manner, over time.

The frequency that pain assessment is required is as individual as the pain itself. It is dependent on:

- the severity of the pain;

- the changing nature of the patient's medical condition;

- the stability of the pain; and

- the effectiveness of current pain control interventions.

Figure 7.4 depicts various pain intensity rating scales, developed to record the severity of pain experienced. These have been shown to be effective patient self-report instruments (McCaffery and Beebe, 1989). The choice of scale will be dependent on patient preference, language and fluency of language spoken, and on ease of reproducibility. Patients have been shown to use a variety of words when describing their pain (Tearnan and Cleeland as cited by Twycross, 1994:144), and this must be kept in mind with the choice of scale.

**Figure 7.4 Pain intensity rating scales**

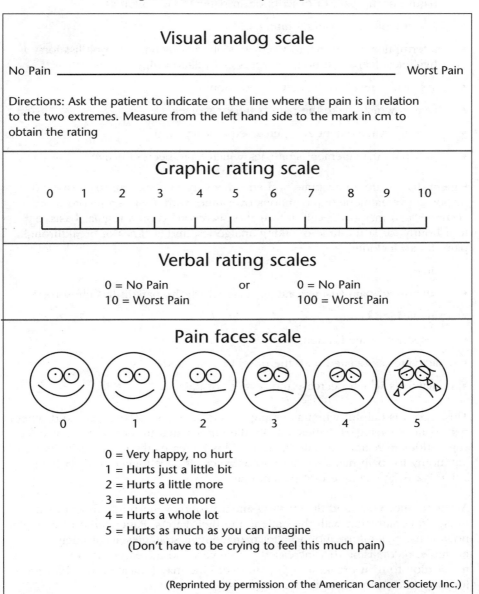

## Visual analog scale

No Pain _____ Worst Pain

Directions: Ask the patient to indicate on the line where the pain is in relation to the two extremes. Measure from the left hand side to the mark in cm to obtain the rating

## Graphic rating scale

0    1    2    3    4    5    6    7    8    9    10

## Verbal rating scales

0 = No Pain          or          0 = No Pain
10 = Worst Pain                  100 = Worst Pain

## Pain faces scale

0          1          2          3          4          5

0 = Very happy, no hurt
1 = Hurts just a little bit
2 = Hurts a little more
3 = Hurts even more
4 = Hurts a whole lot
5 = Hurts as much as you can imagine
    (Don't have to be crying to feel this much pain)

(Reprinted by permission of the American Cancer Society Inc.)

An important factor in the use of these scales is the *constancy* of the scale chosen. There will be a greater likelihood of consistency of patient reports regarding the presence and severity of pain when the patient becomes used to describing their pain in the same manner over time.

Information included in a thorough pain assessment includes:

- time since pain onset;
- site(s) of pain, including radiation;
- nature of the pain (a description in patient's own words);
- severity of pain (using a rating scale);
- interruption/impairment to activities of daily living, e.g. mobilisation, hygiene, sleep, nutrition, interpersonal relationships;
- associated levels of anxiety, depression;
- factors which make the pain better or worse;
- current management and perceived efficacy; and
- past pain management strategies which have been effective.

Patient diaries are an accurate and effective way to track pain patterns and response to treatments/interventions over time, with a written record more accurate than memory recall. Information is recorded on a regular basis, e.g. four hourly, or at the time of taking analgesics, and at times of breakthrough pain. It can include:

- time;
- severity of pain (using a rating scale which the patient has chosen);
- medication taken;
- response to medication;
- activities associated with the onset of pain; and
- activities which decrease the severity of pain.

This record is helpful when assessing the effectiveness of analgesia and other pain control strategies. Patients make the entries and are encouraged to offer suggestions in relation to interventions. This increases their responsibility and autonomy for pain management and enhances independence in daily living. Table 7.2 is an example of a patient diary.

Accurate, thorough, and timely assessment is one of the prime functions of the nurse, in conjunction with the patient and their carers. Patients must be taught how to use this information to alter management strategies accordingly, for example, recognising that increased pain levels and increased use of medication to treat breakthrough pain over time may indicate a need for an increase in dose or strength of analgesics.

**Table 7.2 A patient diary**

| DATE/TIME | SEVERITY OF PAIN Rating scale: 0 = no pain 1 = mild pain 2 = moderate pain 3 = severe pain 4 = worst pain imaginable | PAIN MEDICATION: name of drug dose | ACTIVITIES AT TIME OF PAIN ONSET | PAIN RATING 1 HOUR AFTER TAKING MEDICATION |
|---|---|---|---|---|
| 26/7 7AM | 0 | MS Contin 30mg | | 1 |
| 11AM | 3 | Morphine mixture 2mg/ml – 3ml Panadol x2 | Had a shower | 1 |
| 3PM | 0 | Panadol x2 | | 0 |
| 7PM | 1 | MS Contin 30mg Panadol X2 | Had dinner | 0 |
| 11PM | 2 | Panadol x2 | Going to bed | |

(Adapted from McCaffery and Beebe, 1989:30)

# MULTIDISCIPLINARY PAIN MANAGEMENT

The complexities of cancer pain control require a multidisciplinary approach to provide effective care for the person with cancer pain. Recognising when referrals are required becomes an important part of the nursing role, and is likely to facilitate optimal patient functioning and quality of life.

The medical role in the team is twofold — treatment of the underlying malignancy, and symptom control. Anti-cancer treatments should be considered for all patients with disease-related pain, and this may lead to a reduced need for analgesia and other symptom control measures (Woodruff, 1996:80).

The third case history can serve as an illustration here. Mr Brown will benefit from a home assessment to check for safe access to all areas of his house. Walking aids can provide balance and security. Discussions with a social worker may lead to the initiation of needed community supports, and volunteers may provide both practical help and company. Palliative care services may be required for 24-hour contact for Brian. The role of the patient's general practitioner is also essential for a speedy and appropriate response to changes in the source or severity of pain. Timely referrals can make an enormous difference to coping with long-term illness.

# NURSING ROLES IN PAIN CONTROL

The most important role held by the nurse is that of patient advocate. Implicit in this is an unreserved acceptance of the patient's reports of the presence and severity of pain, and a willingness to actively support them in all discussions regarding pain and pain control strategies. Understanding and knowledge may be the lock to open the door, but attitude is the key. Without a positive attitude towards the priority of pain control, the door to better practice will remain closed.

One must never underestimate the strength of a therapeutic nurse–patient relationship, with its potential to foster a positive and helpful exchange of ideas. Initiating purposeful conversation in relation to the common misconceptions regarding cancer pain provides an opportunity for practical education. Inaccurate ideas can be replaced with truths, and examples from clinical practice can help in the formation of positive patient attitudes. Thorough discharge planning following inpatient admissions will ensure that the patient returns to a safe home environment, with adequate mechanisms in place for ongoing assessment of pain and daily living activities. This is essential, as cancer pain is usually an ongoing problem.

Patient education is paramount. Chronic pain management is a 24-hour responsibility, therefore the patient and their carers must have the knowledge, skills, and confidence to respond quickly to changes in pain. Theoretical and practical teaching of analgesic and non-analgesic methods is a continuing function as long as pain remains a problem.

# PAIN MANAGEMENT: NON-ANALGESIC METHODS

Non-analgesic methods of pain management are likely to enhance the effects of medical treatments. They can often be taught easily to carers, and will provide benefits in relation to independence in pain management. The use of these methods recognises the benefits of a holistic approach to care, based on the interplay of mind, spirit and body (Rankin-Box, 1988).

Non-analgesic approaches will not relieve pain in the manner of analgesics, but will reduce the perception of pain during their application, and for a varied amount of time afterwards. These techniques are not intended to replace analgesic methods; but they should used in conjunction to provide optimal relief. They also help strengthen the nurse–patient relationship through the provision of individualised attention (McCaffery and Beebe, 1989).

Determining which method is most effective is often a matter of trial and error, therefore patients should be encouraged to try a variety of techniques to find those which most suit them. Table 7.3 presents a number of techniques for consideration, with readers encouraged to read McCaffery and Beebe (1989) for further excellent practical information in this area. The methods listed are low-risk, readily available and easy to use, and appropriate for patients with limited energy levels.

**Table 7.3 Non-pharmacologic methods of pain control**

| METHOD OF PAIN CONTROL AND EXAMPLES | DESCRIPTION AND RATIONALE FOR USE | EXPECTED BENEFITS |
|---|---|---|
| Superficial massage e.g. massage of feet, hands, back | Stimulation of the skin <br>• decreases the intensity of pain felt through inhibition of nociceptor activity <br>• may lead to endorphin release <br>• promotes distraction from pain <br>• relieves muscle spasm and promotes general relaxation | • Easy to use and teach <br>• May reduce anxiety <br>• Increased muscle flexibility |
| Application of heat (dry or moist heat) | Applied at a comfortable level of intensity for no longer than 15 minutes <br>• relieves muscle spasm <br>• promotes distraction from pain | • Works best for localised pain <br>• Easy to use and teach |
| Application of cold/ice | • Cold is applied at a comfortable level of intensity for no longer than 30 minutes <br>• Ice is applied directly to the skin for no longer than 10 minutes <br>• Both lead to numbness and desensitisation of peripheral nerve endings | • Works best for localised pain <br>• Temporary pain relief following acute injury <br>• Easy to use and teach |
| Transcutaneous electrical nerve stimulation (TENS) | Application of electrodes to the skin, and generation of a low current <br>• may lead to increased release of endorphins <br>• may reduce the number of pain impulses reaching the CNS through activation of mechanoreceptors | • Works best with localised pain |
| Imagery (linked with distraction) e.g. breathing out pain, ball of healing energy | • Uses the imagination to control pain <br>• May be used to produce an 'image of pain relief' | • Can result in increased tolerance to pain <br>• May be used to produce relaxation |
| Distraction e.g. use of visual concentration and rhythmic massage, slow rhythmic breathing, laughter | Focuses attention on stimuli other than the pain sensation, with pain then becoming on the periphery of awareness | • May lead to an increase in pain tolerance <br>• Works well with brief episodes of pain, e.g. diagnostic procedures |
| Relaxation e.g. meditation, yoga, music, heartbeat breathing, peaceful past experiences | • Engenders a state of freedom from anxiety and skeletal muscle tension <br>• Produces a decrease in activity of the autonomic nervous system | The exact benefits for people in pain remain unknown, but may be related to the interaction between pain, muscle tension, and anxiety |

(Adapted from McCaffery and Beebe, 1989)

# PAIN MANAGEMENT: ANALGESIC METHODS

Analgesics are the most common drugs prescribed for those with cancer, and morphine is the most common opioid analgesic used (Ashby et al., 1992; Curtis and Declan Walsh, 1993). There is a range of analgesics available, therefore an understanding of the different types of drugs used and the rationale behind their choice is required.

Knowledge of the underlying mechanisms of pain leads to a clearer understanding regarding the use of different drugs. Pain classifications are useful tools to guide analgesic (and other methods of) management. The WHO classification describes cancer pain in terms of its intensity. Analgesics of increasing strength are introduced to correlate with these levels of severity (see Figure 7.2) (Twycross, 1994) and can also be given according to the source of the pain stimulus and the structures involved (see Figure 7.3.) Morphine is the opioid analgesic of choice for strong cancer pain (WHO, 1986).

Using a structural approach, analgesics can be classified into those that act mainly within the central nervous system (brain and spinal cord), and those that act mainly at the level of the peripheral nervous system. Table 7.4 presents the commonly used analgesics classified in this way.

The principles guiding the selection of analgesics are consistent with those guiding all symptom control measures: the intervention must be the least disruptive and must contribute to overall quality of life. For this reason, oral administration is the route of choice, and most patients can continue in this way for the entire course of their disease.

It is usual for patients with an ongoing pain problem to be placed on regular doses of an opioid analgesic, in addition to a non-opioid preparation. Slow-release morphine preparations, e.g. MS Contin® or Kapanol®, have the advantage of reducing the number and times of tablet taking. Some studies have shown an increase in compliance with dosing through the use of such preparations (Portenoy et al., 1989; Hiraga et al., 1989). As compliance with ongoing medications has been shown to be a problem (Turk and Rudy, 1991; Sackett et al., 1991), this is an important factor in choice of analgesics.

It will have been noted that no mention has been made of average doses of analgesics. In relation to morphine use, the dose will depend on the patient's previous medications, age, and general condition and, most importantly, pain severity. There is no maximum daily dose for morphine (as a general rule), which is one of the reasons for its widespread use in cancer pain management.

An essential component of analgesic therapy is timely side effects management. Many side effects are dose-related, that is, increasing doses are associated with an increase in the severity of side effects experienced. Some side effects may create such problems that the offending drug may have to be ceased. For example, aspirin can cause gastric irritation and may interfere

## Table 7.4 Analgesics used in cancer pain management

| DRUG CLASSIFICATION AND PREDOMINANT SITE OF ACTION | GENERIC DRUG NAMES (WITH SOME EXAMPLES OF TRADE NAMES) | MECHANISM OF ACTION (RELATED TO PAIN CONTROL) |
|---|---|---|
| **Opioids:**<br>A general term to include all drugs with morphine-like action.<br>Site of action:<br>• central nervous system (CNS)<br>(opioid receptors have been found in nearly all organs) | *Strong opioids:*<br>• morphine (MS Contin®, Kapanol®)<br>• diamorphine (heroin)<br>• methadone (Physeptone®)<br>• pethidine<br>• oxycodone (Proladone®, Endone®)<br>• fentanyl<br>• hydrocodone (Hycomine®)<br>*Weak opioids:*<br>• codeine (component of Panadeine®, Panadeine forte®)<br>• dihydrocodeine (Rikodeine®)<br>• dextropropoxyphene (component of Digesic®)<br>• pentazocine (Fortral®) | • Bind with opioid receptors and block transmission of potentially painful impulses to the CNS<br>• Opioids interact to a variable extent with receptors:<br>• strong binding<br>• weak binding |
| *Non-steroidal anti-inflammatory agents:*<br>Analgesics with anti-inflammatory properties<br>Site of action:<br>• peripheral nervous system | • aspirin (acetylsalicylic acid) (Aspro®, Disprin®)<br>• indomethacin (Indocid®)<br>• ibuprofen (Brufen®, Nurofen®)<br>• naproxen (Naprosyn®) | • Inhibit production of prostaglandins (PGs) (which sensitise nociceptive nerve endings) and other substances released with tissue injury<br>• Reduce inflammation<br>• Reduce peripheral neural sensitisation<br>• Anti-pyretic effects |
| *Steroidal anti-inflammatory agents:*<br>Site of action:<br>• peripheral nervous system | • prednisolone (Delta Cortef®, Solone®)<br>• dexamethasone (Dexmethsone®) | • Reduce inflammation and peripheral neural sensitisation<br>• Reduce excitability of neurons to potentially painful (nociceptive) stimuli |
| **Simple analgesics**<br>Site of action:<br>• central nervous system | • paracetemol (Panadol®, Panamax®) | • Reduction in pain perception through various mechanisms, e.g. reduction in PG production<br>• anti-pyretic action |
| *Agents which reduce skeletal and smooth muscle spasm*<br>Site of action:<br>• peripheral nervous system | • hyoscine (Buscopan®)<br>• peppermint oil<br>• clonidine (Catapres®)<br>• benzodiazepines (diazepam, clonazepam) | • Prevent release of acetyl choline in smooth muscle<br>• Reduce sensitivity of nerves to stimulation in skeletal muscle<br>• Reduce anxiety |

(Adapted from Twycross, 1994)

with platelet formation. These may be unacceptable in a person receiving chemotherapy who already has problems with mucositis and lowered blood counts. Paracetemol may be used as an alternative in this situation.

In case study 1, Mary had an increase in nausea, anorexia and constipation associated with the increase in morphine dose. Treatment of side effects with anti-emetics and aperients led to increased comfort, and assisted with ongoing compliance with analgesics. Diet was monitored to reduce those foods which could be contributing to nausea, and Mary was reassured that most side effects are temporary, and will not be ongoing problems.

**Table 7.5 Side effects of morphine**

| SIDE EFFECT | DEVELOPMENT OF TOLERANCE | DOSE RELATION-SHIP | SOME MANAGEMENT POINTS |
|---|:---:|:---:|---|
| Drowsiness/sedation | ✓ | ✓ | •Warn patients about initial drowsiness, and advise that this problem will lessen over time <br>•Look for contributing factors, e.g. other drugs |
| Nausea and vomiting | ✓ | ✓ | •Use of anti-emetics as required <br>•Small, frequent, low-fat snacks <br>•Advise that this problem will lessen over time |
| Constipation | ✗ | ✓ | •Regular use of a peristaltic stimulant and faecal softener <br>•Encourage fluids |
| Hallucinations/delirium confusion | ✗ | ✓ | •Slow rate of dose increases, or a decrease in dose may be required |
| Myoclonus/agitation | ✗ | ✓ | •Reduce the morphine dose or introduce a benzodiazepine |
| Respiratory depression | ✓ | ✓ | •Use morphine with care in those with obstructive airways disease |
| Physical dependence | ✗ | ✓ | •Slow reduction of dose (if indicated) and maybe concurrent use of benzodiazepine or long-acting opioid, e.g. methadone |

✓ means tolerance does develop to the side effect
✗ means increasing the dose will not lead to a worsening of the side effect

(Adapted from Twycross, 1994)

Table 7.5 presents the major side effects of morphine (the list is not exhaustive), and some important points in relation to its use.

The main principles of analgesic use for chronic cancer pain are outlined as follows:

**R**      regular and round-the-clock dosing

**O**      oral medications if possible

**A**      adjuvants for side effects management

**R**      rescue doses as required for breakthrough pain

**S**      smallest number of medications possible

In those patients for whom the oral route is not possible, the subcutaneous route is often the next least invasive. Infusions can be delivered via a battery-driven syringe driver, such as the Graseby MS16A®, or drug doses can be given intermittently via a butterfly cannula. It must be remembered that not all drugs can be given subcutaneously as they may be irritating to the tissues, and that drug compatibility must be taken into consideration when mixing drugs. The intravenous and intramuscular routes are contraindicated for chronic pain.

Whilst analgesics are seen as one of the major components of pain control, it is believed that the combination of analgesic and non-analgesic methods will provide the best overall pain control, taking into consideration all the components of total pain discussed at the start of this chapter.

# SUMMARY

Cancer pain management presents a challenge to the multidisciplinary team, and often calls for innovative application of many pharmacologic and non-pharmacologic strategies. The role of the nurse is pivotal in effective management, and takes into consideration the multifaceted nature of cancer pain. Positive attitudes will enhance practice, and will be communicated to patients and their carers. Ongoing education will ensure that the patient can take control of pain management, which is essential when pain is a 24-hour problem.

## References

Ashby M, Fleming B, Brooksbank M, Rounsefell B, Runciman W, Jackson K, Muirden N, Smith M (1992): Description of a mechanistic approach to pain management in advanced cancer. *Pain* 51: 153–61.

Brescia F, Portenoy R, Ryan M, Krasnoff L, Gray G (1992): Pain, opioid use, and survival in hospitalised patients with advanced cancer. *Journal of Clinical Oncology* 19 1, January: 149–55.

Casciato D, Lowitz B (eds) (1988): *Manual of Clinical Oncology* (2nd edn). Boston: Little, Brown and Company.

Cleeland C, Gonin R, Hatfield A, Edmonson J, Blum R, Stewart J, Pandya K (1994): Pain and its treatment in outpatients with metastatic cancer. *New England Journal of Medicine* 330, 3 March: 592–596.

Curtis E, Declan Walsh T (1993): Prescribing practices of a palliative care service. *Journal of Pain and Symptom Management* 8 5, July: 312–316.

Foley K (1989): Controversies in cancer pain. *Cancer* 63: 2257–2265.

Hiraga K, Yamamura H, Taguchi T, Takeda F (1989): Clinical Evaluation of Controlled-release Morphine Sulphate Tablets in the Treatment of Cancer Pain. In: Twycross R (ed.): *The Edinburgh Symposium on Pain Control and Medical Education. International Congress and Symposium Series No 149.* London: Royal Society of Medicine Services Ltd.

International Association for the Study of Pain Subcommittee on Taxonomy (1979): *Pain.* 6: 249–52.

McCaffery M, Beebe A (1989): *Pain: Clinical Manual for Nursing Practice.* USA: The CV Mosby Company.

Murphy G, Lawrence W, Lenhard R (eds) (1995): *American Cancer Society Textbook of Clinical Oncology* (2nd edn). USA: The American Cancer Society.

O'Connor L (1997): Aspects of morphine compliance in patients self-dosing for cancer pain control. Master of Public Health thesis, Monash University.

Portenoy R, Maldonado M, Fitzmartin R, Kaiko R, Kanner R (1989): Oral controlled-release morphine sulphate. *Cancer* 63: 2284–88.

Rankin-Box D (ed.)(1988): *Complementary Health Therapies: A Guide for Nurses and the Caring Professions.* Australia: Croom Helm.

Rimer B, Levy M, Keintz M, Fox L, Engstrom P, MacElwee N (1987): Enhancing cancer pain control regimes through patient education. *Patient Education and Counselling* 10: 267–77.

Sackett D, Haynes R, Guyatt G, Tugwell P (1991): *Clinical Epidemiology: A Basic Science for Clinical Medicine* (2nd edn). Boston: Little, Brown and Company.

Turk D, Rudy T (1991): Neglected topics in the treatment of chronic pain patients — relapse, noncompliance, and adherence enhancement. *Pain* 4: 5–28.

Twycross R (1994): *Pain Relief in Advanced Cancer.* Singapore: Churchill Livingstone.

Woodruff R (1996): *Cancer Pain.* Melbourne: Asperula Pty Ltd.

World Health Organisation (1986): *Cancer Pain Relief.* Geneva: World Health Organisation.

# SECTION THREE

## *The challenge: Issues for nurses*

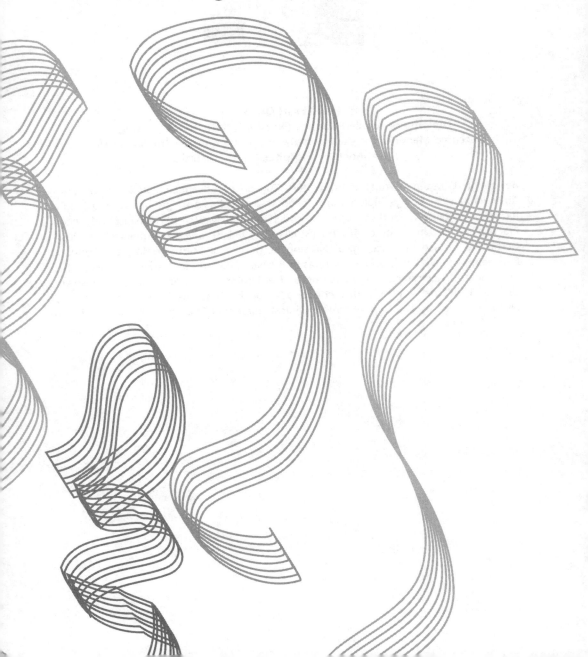

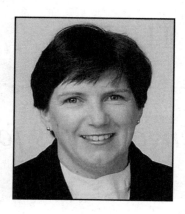

**BEVERLEIGH QUESTED**
**Diploma of Applied Science (Nursing), Bachelor of Nursing**
**Outcome Manager for the Haematology–Bone Marrow Transplant Unit**
**Royal Adelaide Hospital, South Australia**

Beverleigh Quested graduated from Sturt College of Advanced Education in South Australia in 1981 with a Diploma of Applied Science (Nursing). She has since gained a Bachelor of Nursing and is currently undertaking a Master of Nursing (Advanced Practice) at the University of South Australia. In 1983 Beverleigh completed the Post-Certificate Course in Oncological Nursing at the Royal Marsden Hospital, London. Beverleigh has worked in oncology units in Brisbane, London and Adelaide since 1981, with most of her clinical experience on a Haematology and Bone Marrow Transplant Unit. In 1997 she was the course coordinator for the Graduate Diploma in Oncology Nursing offered by The Department of Clinical Nursing at The University of Adelaide in South Australia.

# Chapter 8

## *Assessing and knowing the person with cancer*

This chapter has two central concepts. One is of knowing each individual patient — what they value, how they cope, their physical reactions, and who is important to them. The other concept looks at the 'normal'; how, as Calkin (1984) theorises, novice nurses deal with common responses to a situation, and how, with more experience and expertise, nurses are able to comprehend and care for a wider range of patient responses. As nurses, we fit our patients within the range of our clinical experience. By coming to know our patients better we configure the individual patient and their 'normal' into our clinical experience.

Both of these concepts affect the manner in which patients are assessed by nurses, and the care they receive. The two concepts will be applied to nursing assessment of cancer patients.

## THE NURSE–PATIENT RELATIONSHIP

Oncology nurses (including myself) find it very rewarding to be with and get to know cancer patients well over the months (often years) that they return for treatment and follow-up appointments (Cohen et al., 1994; Steeves et al., 1994). This knowing can be used to recognise problems in and with patients.

The concept of knowing a patient can be thought of as creating a picture, with the brief information obtained at handover and from reading the case notes or referral providing a sketchy outline. As we come to know our patient, the sketch develops into a larger, more detailed picture, with colour and shading. The outlines are more clearly drawn in certain areas, with the patient's social context adding background. The picture is an interpretation of the patient that, as nurses, we make in the context of the nurse–patient relationship. While the picture may never be totally accurate it aids in understanding the patient (Barker, 1987; Radwin, 1995:367).

Tanner et al. (1993: 275) put forward the idea that 'nurses frequently describe knowing the patient as getting a sense of the patient as a person'. 'Swanson (1991) defined knowing as striving to understand an event as it had meaning in the life of the patient' (cited in Radwin, 1996:1142–3).

Knowing the patient is important for nursing practice in four specific ways:

1. patients are recognised and treated as individuals;

2. subtle changes in condition are detected and may improve patient care;

3. clinical judgement and decision-making are enhanced by patient-specific knowledge; and

4. individual patients help develop the nurse's understanding of the larger patient population (Radwin, 1996; Tanner et al., 1993; Evans, 1996:18).

Getting a sense of the patient as a distinct individual and understanding the meaning events have in the patient's life are critical features of knowing the patient and allowing individualisation of care. In practice it is more difficult to care for patients who are new — patient-specific information is not available and simple tasks such as bathing, daily routines and preferred name all have to be established. Knowing the patient means the care of that patient can consider and incorporate the values, hopes, needs and individuality of the patient as a person. Knowing is a concept that takes time for nurses to develop within our practice, because, at first, just completing all the care required by a patient within the shift is a challenge.

Radwin (1996) identified chronological time as one factor that relates to knowing the patient. Cancer care and treatment involves repeated visits and hospitalisations, allowing nurses to build up a vast array of specific patient information. Comparisons can be made between this encounter, previous encounters with this patient and experience with the larger patient population. Nurses spend more time with patients than do other health professionals. Knowing a patient's normal responses, a nurse can detect subtle changes.

Tanner et al. (1993:275) define two broad categories of knowing the patient:

1. Knowing the patient as a person.

2. In-depth knowledge of the patient's pattern of responses including:

   • responses to therapeutic measures;

   • routines and habits;

   • coping resources;

   • physical capabilities and endurance; and

   • body topology and characteristics.

realms provides valuable insights for their ongoing support and care. Such knowledge influences how we provide education to our patients, how we support them as they cope with their disease and how we plan for their discharge.

Social aspects for assessment include an awareness of the important people in our patient's life, our patient's living arrangements and what supports they need and receive. Patients undergoing cancer treatment move through a variety of treatment settings from hospital to outpatient departments to home care. Prompt discharge with short-as-possible stays are a feature of health care administration in the current economic climate so more patients are being managed in the community. Discharge planning starts on admission to hospital, but all areas of the health care system need to liaise to ensure appropriate community support, therefore an understanding of the patient's life outside of hospital is needed. Some areas for consideration include:

- How has the illness affected their social role and function? Can they still work, care for their children, pets or aging parents? Consider shopping/financial/transport/living arrangements. What was their pre-hospital routine?

- Who are the important people in their lives? Who brings them to hospital? Who visits them and how often? Who provides what type of support? Consider family, friends, church or social groups. What community supports does the patient have and what is available?

- Can they carry out essential activities of daily living such as dressing, bathing and eating? How well are they cared for? Do they need and want help; if so, what type and how often? Where does the patient live, in an urban or rural setting? Can they leave their home unaided?

- Can they administer their own medication and treatment regimes? What is their literacy and educational level (to ensure appropriate client learning and comprehension)? Consider the main caregivers and include the patient and the carer(s) when providing education and planning for the patient's discharge.

- What cultural issues affect their understanding of their disease and care?

- How have they coped with problems in the past? Do they use denial or become depressed?

- How has the disease and its treatment affected them? How do they feel about this? What bothers them most about the treatment and/or the disease?

It has been well documented that patients and families who have an increased knowledge of their illness and treatment plan experience significantly less anxiety and stress than those who do not (Cornelius, 1994:625). In view of this, when patients are discharged they need contact numbers of either the ward, the general practitioner, the consultant or the health care agency to prevent

The overall skin colour of the patient is an obvious and easily noted physiognomic characteristic. Skin colour deviations suggest compromises in metabolism, circulation or oxygenation (Fuller and Schaller-Ayres, 1994:131). Normal skin is warm, intact, and well perfused; changes can be compared to the patient's normal colour and to that of the larger population group. Yellow tinges to the skin can be subtle or dramatic, and can be due to impaired bilirubin metabolism through liver dysfunction or through excessive red cell destruction. Jaundice in some populations may be detectable only by ascertaining the colour of the eye sclera. Pale skin colour is seen in a low haemoglobin concentration, and can be due to deficiency (anaemia) or to physiological causes such as peripheral shutdown. A generalised redness can be the body's attempt to control temperature by systemic vasodilatation or it can be part of an inflammatory response, for example, in graft versus host disease or antibiotic sensitivity. Localised redness may be due to local inflammatory response, radiotherapy treatment or radiation recall reactions. Confirmation from the patient will help in deciding which is the most likely. Cyanosis results from decreased oxygen-carrying haemoglobin and can be central, or peripheral, which may be the result of restricted blood flow and subsequent oxygen level reduction to an area. Most nurses can detect these changes easily in acute presentations, but knowing patients allows detection to occur earlier.

One common side effect of radiotherapy and chemotherapy is myelosuppression. Because bone marrow cells divide rapidly they can be affected by chemotherapy and radiotherapy which act on cell division. Bone marrow can also be invaded by metastatic cancer cells that physically crowd out normal blood cell production. Problems with myelosuppression include an increased tendency to bleed and a decreased ability to fight infections. Both of these problems can have dire consequences, and because of this, oncology nurses focus a great deal on detecting and preventing problems in these areas.

The position, type, size, colour and cause of a bruise can provide an insight into pathophysiological processes occurring, and can trigger further investigation of the patient's haematological state. Bruises are the result of extravasation of blood from a vessel into tissue. Bleeding is stopped by vasoconstriction, formation of a platelet plug and the activation of clotting factors that cause fibrin clot formation (Gaspard, 1994). The position and size of the bruises can provide some clues as to the patient's condition. Some bruises occur as a direct result of trauma (the patient accidentally knocks themselves); other bruises occur spontaneously as the result of small tears in vessel walls. The size of a bruise can reflect the amount of trauma caused and/or the pathophysiology of the patient. Bruises caused by a low platelet count happen quickly and usually involve skin and mucous membranes; blood continues to leak out of the vessel until sufficient platelets can form a platelet plug. Problems with reduced clotting factors result in deeper bruising over a longer time, as the platelet plug initially reduces blood extravasation but is unable to be stabilised, resulting in further bleeding. In some patients there may be problems with both clot formation and coagulation, leaving them very vulnerable to haemorrhage.

Bruises are classified as to the size and type of the tissue involved. **Petechiae** are small bruises 1–3 mm and occur in the normal population in response to superficial skin damage. In oncology patients, who have a low platelet count, petechiae can occur on the fronts of shins from the sheer pressure of walking, or can be caused by tight clothing or tourniquets. Other types of bruises are **purpura** which are larger than petechiae and pink to purple in colour; **ecchymoses** which are purple to green to yellow and then brown over time, and **haematoma,** which is a collection of blood in the deeper tissues. The colour of the bruise reflects the breakdown of red cell components in the body tissues (Fuller and Schaller-Ayres, 1996).

Blood loss from nose bleeds, continued oozing from puncture sites, haematuria, heavy loss through menstruation, and rectal bleeding are common and need to be investigated because small consistent losses can be substantial over time. A low platelet count may be the most significant factor for bleeding in oncology patients (Groenwald et al., 1997). Investigating the patient for altered clotting function or low platelets may reveal one of the reasons for the blood loss.

A nurse touching a patient's skin can get some idea as to the patient's state. All nurses have at some stage touched a patient, thought the patient felt hot and confirmed with a thermometer, or replaced a thermometer because the nurse believed the patient to be hotter than the thermometer indicated. Temperatures are thought to be a protective mechanism — when core temperature is raised the invading pathogen is prevented from reproducing as easily (Porth, 1994:180). Knowing the patient helps the nurse decide whether to administer paracetamol to reduce a fever. Some patients will resist taking the drug, as it makes them uncomfortable, they sweat profusely and in a short time their temperature rebounds higher through rigoring. Rigors increase the body's metabolic rate but the muscle action produces little work so all the energy goes into heat production thus increasing the body's temperature.

Temperatures can also be a symptom of paraneoplastic processes. The pattern of fevers or the correlations of increased heart rate with fever or with the timing of fevers during the day may provide some insight into the cause of the temperature rise as part of a disease or infective process. Up to 30–45 per cent of temperatures in cancer patients are not infection related (Groenwald et al., 1997), however fever remains the most reliable indicator of infection in a myelosuppressed patient (Haeuber and Spross, 1994:382). Knowing the patient helps in determining possible causes of fever.

When the immune system has been compromised the normal signs and symptoms of infection such as redness and swelling are reduced. Pus contains dead white cells. The myelosuppressed patient has few white cells so pus formation may be absent or substantially reduced (LaRocco, 1994:248–249). Fever is the most reliable indicator of infection but, as discussed, can be problematic. Sources of infection need to be checked and isolated. The most obvious sites of infection in the oncology patient are the skin, the respiratory tract and the gastrointestinal and urinary tracts (Haeuber and Spross, 1994:383).

Open wounds are also potential sites for infection, as are central venous catheters or subcutaneous lines. Ulceration is possible with skin metastasis but can also be due to chemotherapy extravasation, radiation treatment and pressure sores. Metastatic skin infiltrates occur in lung, breast, lymphoma and squamous cell carcinomas of the head and neck occasionally but are possible with many cancer types (Couillard-Getneur and Heery, 1994:428). Abnormal bulges, lumps and breaks need to be investigated as to their cause and the implications for the patient. Nodules, lumps and painful spots can alert us to finding a cause — is this a recurrence or an infiltrate?

Scars provide evidence of previous surgery and procedures such as central line insertions or node biopsy. The presence of implanted devices such as infusaports can be detected by asking the patient, looking for insertion scars, and palpating for the device under the skin. A note of caution with implanted devices is that ports can be used for intrathecal, arterial and venous access, so before needling or using the device, the vessel in which it is implanted should be identified. Radiotherapists use small tattoos for mapping radiotherapy fields. Skin dryness may be affected by dehydration, by drugs, by graft versus host disease or, occasionally, by local radiotherapy reactions.

Skin texture, thickness, elasticity, mobility, and fat deposition are indicators of weight loss, nutrition and hydration. Inadequate intake will lead to the utilisation of stored fat as an energy source and when this is expended muscle tissue will be used. The presence and placement of fat stores on the body and evidence of muscle wasting indicate the level of fat and protein stores. Malnutrition is a crucial issue for many patients, stemming from psychological factors such as body image (due to cachexia) and physical factors related to disease throughout the intestinal tract.

Hair loss is one of the most known side effects of cancer treatment and one which concerns patients initially, and requires an adjustment of their self-concept and body image. The presence or absence of hair and the amount of growth may provide a clue to the recent treatment of a patient. A telltale sign in many oncology patients is the presence of beanies, scarves, turbans and various hats to prevent heat loss due to the volume of blood flow that the scalp receives.

Finally, is the patient clean and well cared for or dishevelled? This may be a personal choice but it provides some insight into living conditions, family support and the ability to care for oneself. Social and cultural choices are reflected in the manner of dress and adornment of the body, for example, tattoos or body piercing. Observing the patient's skin provides many insights into the social, cultural and physical dimensions of a patient.

To return to the picture metaphor, the evolving picture is now drawn with a depth of structure, colour, texture and detail, including the interrelationship between patient and family and the meanings of illness, disease, symptoms and care. The patient is placed within a network of people; a patient context outside of the hospital environment has been added. The picture will continue to evolve as more areas are assessed. With each encounter another layer is added, providing further dimensions for the nurse's constructed image of the patient.

# CONCLUSION

Knowing the patient means considering the patient as a person as well as the biophysical object. Knowing the patient allows us as nurses to understand the patient's normal life, including their past and their present, and, through assessment, to plan and predict the patient's future care. When assessing, nurses appear to structure the importance of information and combination of information with comparisons of what is expected in similar patients or with constructs specific to the patient in question (Crow et al., 1995). Assessment is the first step in the nursing process. Clinical judgement is needed to consider the accumulated data, discard irrelevant information, retain the important points and then identify and prioritise patient problems (Grossman et al., 1996). The expert does this seamlessly, integrating small isolated facts into a broad picture. We all think in differing ways, however recognising the significance of information and drawing conclusions from the information are fundamental processes.

Benner and Wrubel (1982) describe nurses who developed their clinical knowledge by studying patient data, listing it, writing it down, discussing it with colleagues and keeping records of when their clinical assessment and judgement were right and when they were wrong. The use of reflection on practice enables some of the assumptions, developments and progression in practice to be explored. How individual nurses cognitively do this is not fully understood; that we do it is recognised and is sometimes called intuition (Benner and Tanner, 1987).

How do we decide what is important? How do we develop a sense of salience? Below are some of the questions that I consider are important to ask in deciding the priority of care:

- What is life threatening?

- What bothers the patient the most?

- What could be potentially life threatening?

- What is readily fixed?

- What has to be done first because of information or institutional needs?

As nurses, we spend the most time with patients; we have the best opportunity to identify problems in relation to individual patients by observing subtle qualitative changes. As nurses, we need to acknowledge and value the contextual knowledge that we gather from our patients. Clinical nurses ground their practice in both experience and theoretical knowledge. When we know our patients our assessments can incorporate all areas of knowledge in order to ensure an optimal outcome for each patient.

This chapter may seem to contain material that is simple, obvious and common sense. It is nevertheless one attempt to articulate and acknowledge the subtle finesse and astute skill of the nurse that comes from experience and expertise in caring for and getting to know patients. The acquisition of clinical experience is a gradual process, often not noticed along the way. It becomes taken for granted when it should be recognised, claimed and valued as part of the unique skill of nurses.

# References

Barker P (1987): Assembling the pieces. *Nursing Times* 25 November 83 47: 67–68.

Benner P, Tanner C (1987): Clinical judgement: How expert nurses use intuition. *American Journal of Nursing* 87: 23–31.

Benner P, Wrubel J (1982): Skilled clinical knowledge: The value of perceptual awareness. *Nurse Educator* 7: 11–17.

Benner P, Wrubel J (1989): *The Primacy of Caring: Stress and Coping in Health and Illness.* Menlo Park: Addison-Wesley.

Calkin JD (1984): A model for advanced nursing practice. *The Journal of Nursing Administration* 14 1: 24–30.

Cohen M, Haberman E, Steeves R, Deatrick J (1994): Rewards and difficulties of oncology nursing. *Oncology Nursing Forum* supplement 21 8: 9–17.

Cornelius F (1994): Home Care and Alternative Care Settings and Cancer Resources. In: Otto SE: *Oncology Nursing.* St Louis: Mosby, pp. 611–640.

Coulliard-Getreuer DL, Heery ML (1994): Skin. In: Gross J, Johnson BL (eds): *Handbook of Oncology Nursing.* Boston: Jones and Bartlett, pp. 421–463.

Coyle N, Goldstein ML, Passik S, Fishman B, Portenoy R (1996): Development and validation of a patient needs assessment tool (PNAT) for oncology clinicians. *Cancer Nursing* 19 2: 81–92.

Crow RA, Chase J, Lamond D (1995): The cognitive component of nursing assessment: An analysis. *Journal of Advanced Nursing* 22: 206–212.

Evans L (1996): Knowing the patient: The route to individualized care. *Journal of Gerontological Nursing* 22 3: 15–19.

Fuller J, Schaller-Ayres J (1994): *Health Assessment: A Nursing Approach* (2nd edn). Philadelphia: J.B. Lippincott.

Gaspard KJ (1994): Alterations in Hemostasis. In: Porth CM: *Pathophysiology Concepts of Altered Health States*. Philadelphia: J.B. Lippincott, pp. 311–320.

Groenwald SL, Frogge MH, Goodman M, Yarbro CH (1997): *Cancer Nursing Principles and Practice* (4th edn). Boston: Jones and Bartlett.

Grossman S, Campbell C, Riley B (1996): Assessment of clinical decision-making ability of critical care nurses. *Dimensions of Critical Care Nursing* 15 5: 272–278.

Haeuber D, Spross J (1994): Bone Marrow. In: Gross J, Johnson BL (eds): *Handbook of Oncology Nursing*. Boston: Jones and Bartlett, pp. 373–399.

LaRocco M (1994): Inflammation and Immunity. In: Porth CM: *Pathophysiology Concepts of Altered Health States*. Philadelphia: J.B. Lippincott, pp. 243–264.

Mallett J, Bailey C (1996): *The Royal Marsden NHS Trust Manual of Clinical Procedures* (4th edn). Oxford: Blackwell Science.

McCarthy MM (1981): The nursing process: Application of current thinking in clinical problem solving. *The Journal of Advanced Nursing* 6: 173–177.

Miaskowski CA, Nielsen B (1985): A cancer nursing assessment tool. *Oncology Nursing Forum* 12 6: 37–42.

Nightingale F (1969): *Notes on Nursing*. New York: Dover Publications.

Porth CM (1994): *Pathophysiology Concepts of Altered Health States*. Philadelphia: J.B. Lippincott.

Radwin L (1995): Knowing the patient: A process model for individualized interventions. *Nursing Research* 44 6: 364–370.

Radwin L (1996): 'Knowing the patient': A review of research on an emerging concept. *Journal of Advanced Nursing* 23: 1142–1146.

Steeves R, Cohen M, Wise C (1994): An analysis of critical incidents describing the essence of oncology nursing. *Oncology Nursing Forum* supplement 21 8: 19–25.

Tanner CA, Benner P, Chesla C, Gordon D (1993): The phenomenology of knowing the patient. *Image: Journal of Nursing Scholarship* 25 4: 273–280.

Tripp-Reimer T (1984): Reconceptualizing the construct of health: Integrating emic and etic perspectives. *Research in Nursing and Health* 7: 101–109.

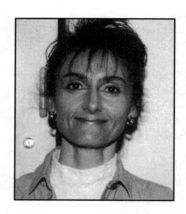

**LOUISE NICHOLSON**
**Master of Nursing, Bachelor of Health Science (Nursing),**
**Oncology Certified Nurse, USA**
**Bone Marrow Transplant Co-ordinator, Department of Medical Oncology**
**Royal Hobart Hospital, Tasmania, Australia**

Louise Nicholson completed her general nursing course at the Royal Children's Hospital in Melbourne in 1984. She has a mixture of oncology nursing experience gained in both paediatric and adult settings including the Prince of Wales Children's Hospital in New South Wales and the Paediatric Oncology and Bone Marrow Transplant Unit of the Memorial Sloan-Kettering Cancer Center in Manhattan, New York.

Between 1989 and 1996 Louise was the Clinical Nurse Consultant at the WP Holman Clinic in Hobart. Recently she was appointed Bone Marrow Transplant Co-ordinator within the Department of Medical Oncology at Royal Hobart Hospital.

The holder of the American credential Oncology Certified Nurse (OCN) Louise has recently completed her Master of Nursing. In the near future Louise would like to undertake her PhD in nursing with the focus being within oncology clinical practice.

# Chapter 9

## *Caring*

## BACKGROUND

Caring as a research topic has held the interest of many nurse researchers since the 1970s. Benner (1984), Roach (1984), Gaut (1984), Watson (1985), Leininger (1985), Larson, P. (1987, 1995), Benner and Wrubel (1988, 1989), Cohen and Sarter (1992), Larson, D. (1992) and Cohen, Haberman and Steeves (1994b) all claim that caring as a phenomenon within the practice of nursing has a major influence and impact on health and illness outcomes through nurse–patient interactions.

Forrest (1989) identified three perspectives of caring:

1. The philosophical perspective developed by Roach (1984) claims that the attributes of compassion, competence, conscience, commitment and confidence are the basis of caring in nursing.
2. Watson's (1985) psychological perspective proposes that caring in nursing is both an art and a science.
3. The anthropological perspective of caring identified by Leininger (1985) examines the cultural differences in the meaning, nature and expression of care.

In Benner and Wrubel's 1989 description, caring is defined as setting up the condition that something or someone outside the person matters, which creates personal concerns. Care sets up a world and creates meaningful distinctions and it is these concerns that provide motivation and direction for people.

Benner (1984) claims that caring cannot be coerced; it can only be understood and facilitated, with caring being embedded in the personal and cultural meanings and commitments of people.

Traditionally, nursing's vision of caring was based in altruism which focused on the nonjudgmental acceptance of the patient and family. However, Nygren's (1935) interpretation of caring (cited in Green-Hernandez, 1991) involves moving beyond altruism, in that caring in nursing combines theological and philosophical notions of caring in its most basic, human expression of shared fellowship. Nurse caring interweaves the therapeutics of healing, helping, empathy and social support in caring for the patient (Green-Hernandez, 1991). This meaning does not derive merely from isolated caring actions. Rather, it emerges from the entire caring process itself.

In Ray's (1988) philosophical analysis of caring, caring is described as being the dominant intellectual, theoretical, heuristic and central practice focus of nursing. This analysis claims there has been no other profession which is so totally concerned with caring behaviors, caring processes and caring relationships.

A review of nursing literature by Gaut (1984) validates two major assumptions regarding the very special place caring has in nursing discourse. The first assumption is that caring is nursing's heritage that nursing's traditions are firmly rooted in the value of care. The second assumption is that caring is a crucial and vital component of nursing.

Gaut (1983, cited in Sherwood, 1991) suggests that in caring there is an action component and an intention. Gaut claims that while the action includes setting goals, choosing tactics to meet goals, and implementing these tactics with skill, the action must be done with the intention of producing positive changes in the patient (Sherwood, 1991).

Gardner (1992) states that the caring dimension of nursing helps to establish the independent practice area of nursing and the growth in professionalism endows caring with a strength that did not exist when it was viewed as a weak form of occupational behaviour. Gardner (1992) claims that, if it is accepted that caring is essential and central to nursing, then it follows that nursing's primary attention should be focused on the practice, study and teaching of caring within nursing. Gardner (1992) has adopted nine assumptions which she states are necessary for the development of caring within nursing. These assumptions are:

1.      Caring is a central and unifying dimension of nursing.
2.      Caring is essential for human growth.
3.      Caring is universally experienced.
4.      Caring is expressed differently within cultures.
5.      Caring behaviours can be learned.
6.      Self-caring is an antecedent to caring for others.

7.      Caring as a necessary and sufficient activity may be separate from or may be associated with curing.

8.      Caring can be categorised in subconstructs.

9.      Caring can be scientifically studied (Gardner, 1992:251).

Several studies have highlighted the importance of caring within oncology nursing. In Mayer's (1986) study cancer care is acknowledged as becoming more complex due to the advances in treatment. However, Mayer claims that because of this there is a concomitant need to maintain humanistic high-touch care, that is, the nontechnical aspect of providing care. Mayer describes five important caring behaviours identified by oncology nurses and says that a caring nurse is one who:

1.      Listens to patients.

2.      Expresses feelings fully about the patient's disease and treatment but treats the information confidentially.

3.      Realises that the patient knows himself or herself the best and, whenever possible, includes the patient in the planning and management of his or her care.

4.      Touches the patient when the patient needs comforting.

5.      Perceives the patient's needs and plans and acts accordingly, for example, gives antinausea medication when the patient is receiving medication that will probably induce nausea.

Larson (1987), Oberle and Davis (1992), and Deatrick and Fischer (1994), in their studies, produced similar results to Mayer's (1986) study. Oberle and Davis (1992) proposed a model of supportive care which identified four dimensions as being necessary for support and caring to occur in a nurse–patient relationship. One of these dimensions was identified as connecting with the patient, which means forming a bond with the patient. This concept of connecting was also identified by Clayton et al. (1991) whose description defined connecting as being a transpersonal experience of feelings that lead to the sense of connection, attachment or bonding between a nurse and a patient and the patient's family.

Benner and Wrubel (1989) identified that the concept of caring in oncology nursing can have a direct influence on the way in which patients make decisions about their care and treatment. Influencing factors included the nurse's demeanor, the tone of the nurse's voice and the questions being answered directly by the nurse. Thus the nurse can have a direct effect on the patient and the patient's family.

The term 'being with' has been identified amongst oncology nurses who have participated in caring studies. One such study was conducted by Haberman et al. (1994) where the caring behaviour of 'being with' was repeatedly described by the nurses as a core concept of oncology nursing. Haberman et al. identified 34 key role dimensions of practice and caring behaviours performed by oncology nurses, which represented the caring behaviours that oncology nurses exhibit and the ways that nurses make a difference in the lives of people with cancer.

In Cohen and Sarter's (1992) exploration of oncology nurses and the meaning of their work, the nurses identified 'being there' for people in the most private moments of suffering and responding to these emotions and needs as important aspects of a caring relationship. Steeves et al. (1994) described 'being there' for patients, 'being with' dying patients and becoming part of the patient's family as important concepts in oncology nursing practice. Cohen et al. (1994a) noted that 'being there' within a patient–nurse relationship produced a form of reward in relation to the action of caring.

## MY STUDY

The purpose of the study I conducted was to further explore and gain understanding of the phenomenon of caring within the practice of oncology nursing. In order to capture the essence of caring, narratives were collected from nurses who care for cancer patients and interpreted to identify the many meanings, concepts and themes which are attached to nurse–patient caring interactions.

The methodology chosen to explore such concepts was through the interpretive paradigm utilising Martin Heidegger's (1927, 1962) hermeneutical phenomenology. Heidegger sought to discover the fundamental meaning of being-in-the-world and attempts to gain access to the world from the human experience through reflection and thematic understanding of the experience.

Through examining day-to-day experiences, Heidegger seeks to expose some of the possible meanings of being. Gullickson (1993) states that Heidegger challenged the dichotomy of subject and object through his need to uncover the meaning of what it is to be human and his recognition of the need of a philosophy which would uncover the meanings of everyday lived experiences. The goal of phenomenological research (Gullickson, 1993) is to understand and discover new meanings that have gone unrecognised because of their perceived everydayness.

According to descriptions from the participants involved in Appleton's (1993) study, the nurse way of 'being there' in caring describes the nurse who centres nursing on the whole person from a humanistic perspective, feels compassion for the person in need and becomes personally involved in helping through caring.

This notion of 'being' in nursing is closely related to Heidegger's (1927, 1962) concept of 'being' which examines the meaning of what it is to be a human being in everyday existence, and the importance that caring and/or concern has to our existence. The nurse's involvement described by Appleton (1993) reveals a sincere, genuine and authentic concern for the patient which develops into more than a professional working relationship. This authentic concern for the patient characterises the nurse's way of 'being there' in caring. By 'being with' patients through empathy, intuition, respect and trust the nurse co-creates a simultaneity and harmony that characterises the nature of helping through intentionally coming to know the person of the patient (Appleton, 1993).

Many of the words, phrases and statements described by McFarlane (1976), Leininger (1984, 1988), Roach (1984), Wolf (1986), Bevis (1988), Watson (1988), Valentine (1989), Sherwood (1991), Gardner (1992) and Donoghue (1993) were identified and acknowledged by the participants involved in the study I conducted. The nurses in my study indicated that empathy, support, improved patient health outcomes, faith, hope, self-actualisation, trust, listening, comforting, honesty, touch, sensitivity, concern and compassion were representative of important caring behaviours in nursing.

Fifteen themes were identified by the nurses participating in my study which represent the caring behaviours that oncology nurses exhibit and the ways that nurses make a difference in the lives of people with cancer. These themes are:

1. Establishing relationships

2. Providing comfort

3. Assisting in decision-making

4. Administering patient treatments

5. Supporting

6. Alleviating suffering

7. Managing pain

8. Maintaining patient privacy

9. Empowering patients/families

10. Dealing with ethical issues

11. Anticipating patients' needs

12. 'Being with'

13. Conveying acceptance

14. Sharing self

15. Encouraging interdisciplinary teamwork.

## Establishing relationships

The oncology nurses put great emphasis on the development and maintenance of the relationship between themselves and the patient and/or the patient's family. The nurses felt these relationships had a positive effect on the patients' health and illness outcomes.

Phrases such as *'getting to know the patient'*, *'becoming involved or attached to patients'*, *'becoming close to patients'* and *'the development of personal interactions with the patient'* were all identified as being important components in the formation of relationships. One nurse said *'caring means forming a friendship with all patients'* while another participant stated *'caring is a reverse process; in order for caring to work the patient must care about the nurse, as well the nurse must care about the patient'*. This was followed by a description which stated *'it is the depth of the patient's needs which will build the nurse–patient relationship'*.

## Providing comfort

Comfort was identified as something the nurses wanted to do to ease the patient's discomfort. This included the physical sense where there was pain from the disease itself, or psychological pain which was caused by anxiety and overwhelming situations. Such descriptions included *'caring comes from the nurse who feels she wants to help relieve the patient's pain, discomfort etc.'*, *'listening and talking to patients'*, *'allaying patients' anxiety'*, *'easing emotional upheavals'* and *'tending to patients' needs'*. One nurse in her description of comfort stated *'caring is doing everything for the patient when they are unable to do it themselves; this makes the patient feel more comfortable, this improves their sense of well being. Finally, caring is providing comfort to patients and their families'*. The use of touch was also acknowledged by one nurse as being a method to provide comfort to cancer patients. She stated *'touching is important in caring, knowing when to touch and when not'*.

## Assisting in decision-making

This was a theme described as being an essential part of the professional nursing role in caring for cancer patients. One nurse stated *'caring involves assisting patients to make decisions'*. Many phrases described this theme including *'providing patients with the opportunity to ask questions'*, *'providing feedback'*, *'being an advocate for the patient'*, *'listening and talking to patients'* and *'being open and direct to patients' questions'*.

## Administering patient treatments

This theme was based on the clinical component of the oncology nurses' practice, with competence and perfection being highlighted within this study as an essential requirement of caring for cancer patients. Statements included *'I need to be an expert in my clinical skills, this will display my competence to the patients I care for'*, *'clinical experience is important in caring for oncology patients'*, *'oncology patients expect perfection from oncology nurses when receiving cancer treatment'* and *'by displaying competence to the patient's families it shows them you care about their loved one'*.

These statements emphasise the importance oncology nurses place on the

# Chapter 10

## *Ethical challenges for cancer nurses*

> *The significant problems we face cannot be solved at the*
> *same level of thinking we were at when we created them*
> *— Albert Einstein*

## INTRODUCTION

The study of morals and ethics can be referred to as a lofty pursuit of philosophers and academics. However, by its nature, the discussion of ethical practice is an activity that all people need to contribute to and participate in. The main objective of ethical inquiry for the health care professions should be to guide judgments in line with what are determined to be sound ethical behaviours, and to provide high-quality care.

The move towards the professionalisation of nursing and the increasing complexity of the health care system in the later part of this century has seen the study of ethics become an integral component of undergraduate and postgraduate nursing education. In 1993, a Code of Ethics was developed by Australian nurses. Its purposes are to:

*   identify the fundamental moral commitments of the profession;
*   provide nurses with a basis for professional and self reflection and a guide to ethical practice; and
*   indicate to the community the values which nurses hold.

Because of this level of education and professional commitment, nurses are now more mindful of the ethical difficulties that arise in their practice. Most nurses would agree that ethical issues continue to be one of the major sources of conflict within the health care team.

It has been suggested that contemporary nursing ethics has held a bias towards analysing what nurses ought to do (ethical judgments), and not enough emphasis has been placed on how nurses themselves should be (ethical behaviour). That is, practitioners need to consider their conduct and integrity as well as their obligations and duties (Tunna and Conner, 1993). How nurses respond and react to ethical difficulties in their practice is as significant as doing the 'right' thing.

Through the presentation of a case study discussion, this chapter will illustrate some of the ethical questions that cancer nurses might need to consider. In addition, the chapter will also focus on the ethical behaviours of nurses, and will identify some of the skills that practitioners need to develop in order to achieve solutions to ethical issues in their practice.

# ETHICAL DILEMMAS AND ETHICAL PROBLEMS

## Ethical dilemmas

By definition a 'dilemma' has no right solution, one can only work towards a resolution. An ethical dilemma occurs when there is a conflict between different moral principles or duties. Therefore, in any given situation, neither principle nor duty can be chosen without violating the other. For example, nurses working with a terminally ill patient faced with the decision to withdraw food and fluids will often experience an ethical dilemma. The dilemma results from a conflict between the moral principles of sanctity of life and non-maleficence on the one hand, and quality of life and beneficence on the other.

Ethical dilemmas obviously do arise in nursing practice, but they are not a common occurrence for the vast majority of practitioners. While the more dramatic ethical dilemmas — such as requests for termination of life, abortion, withdrawal of treatment and other difficult life-and-death decisions — gain a lot of media and public attention they represent only a small proportion of the total of all ethical issues encountered by health care professionals. Most of the ethical challenges that practitioners face every day are problems that occur frequently and are not as visible as the kinds of dilemmas described above. Ethical problems in contrast to ethical dilemmas are more common, less complex and, if analysed carefully, may turn out to be resolvable.

## Ethical problems

Ethical problems usually have solutions, or possible solutions. However, this does not mean that they are less stressful or less difficult to deal with than ethical dilemmas.

Ethical problems can occur because of new or unfamiliar situations, but more often than not they tend to be recurring, unaddressed problems. The following represent a few examples of the questions that cancer nurses ask when confronted by common ethical problems:

- 'Has anyone discussed this with the patient or the family?'

- 'Why won't the doctors listen to me when I try to tell them that the patient does not understand what he has consented for?'

- 'Does anyone know what the doctor told Mrs X and her family about the test results, because she is now sitting on her bed in tears?'

- 'Did the doctor document that NFR [not for resuscitation] order in the patient's notes?'

- 'What does it mean when the doctor writes in the notes "for active management but not for CPR [cardio-pulmonary resuscitation]"?'

Every nurse will be able to identify with these sorts of questions, questions that constitute ethical problems. Nurses faced with familiar ethical problems like these often see them as unresolvable dilemmas. But if these situations were examined more closely, the underlying problems might be seen to result from more practical, resolvable issues. For example, it is not necessarily an ethical dilemma when a doctor has not properly discussed or documented a NFR order. But it does raise an ethical problem that in most institutions would be considered a breach of policy. The nurse has a responsibility to bring the breach of policy, and its implications for patient care, to the attention of the treating doctor.

Problems of poor communication, inadequate explanation, misinterpretation of information or a lack of adherence to policy and procedures are the causes of many day-to-day ethical problems occurring in health care settings.

# BARRIERS TO INTERDISCIPLINARY ETHICAL DECISION-MAKING

Each professional group represented in the health care team undertakes extensive training and education in a particular field that focuses on achieving quality health care outcomes for individuals. However, it does need to be recognised that, frequently, decision-making in health care falls into the ethical arena. The ability to reach a decision that everyone can accept will be dependent on the contribution of each of the groups and disciplines represented in the health care team.

One of the barriers preventing effective interdisciplinary ethical decision-making from taking place has been the hierarchical constitution of the health professions, in which doctors have been seen traditionally as the ultimate decision-makers. There has been an unequal distribution of power, authority and expectation between the role of doctor and the role of nurse at this level of decision-making. Many difficulties arise because the person with the authority to make the decision is not always the same one implementing it. Whilst someone has to take ultimate responsibility for decisions, medical training does not necessarily provide doctors with the knowledge, or the skills, to assume moral authority in ethical decisions. However, this barrier cannot be attributed solely to the authoritative image that the doctor holds within the health care team. Part of it is the problem of powerlessness that is accepted by nurses, who fear the responsibility of facilitating a problem-solving approach themselves towards solving ethical problems.

Nurses must be proactive in initiating debate around ethical issues, and in facilitating the development of problem-solving partnerships with their professional colleagues.

Another reason why nurses find themselves in conflict over ethical issues is the changes in dominant values that have occurred over recent years. One particular value that has been challenged is the concept of paternalism. In the past, a paternalistic outlook created attitudes such as 'the doctor/nurse knows what is best for the patient'. Today, paternalism has been replaced by other core values such as respect for autonomy and patient rights. Where once certain values could be relied on to command general support, for example, the sanctity of life, today these values are being challenged. With continual changes to our value systems, both professionally and personally, there is little wonder that ethical difficulties and conflicts arise.

## Communication

A common complaint amongst nurses is the lack of opportunity to debate ethical issues openly, and to work through a process of decision-making in an appropriate time frame.

For this to be addressed, it is imperative that a common moral ground is established between the different professional groups, and appropriate channels of communication are created to allow interdisciplinary discussion to occur. This process must provide the opportunity for open, honest discussions and should encourage the recognition and acceptance of different professional and personal values. To achieve this, there is an urgent need for practitioners to develop skills that will enable them to participate effectively in constructive and conciliatory processes. Therefore, nurses will need to develop communication, negotiation and mediation skills of a higher order so that they can begin to resolve the many ethical problems that confront them. Mediation is an important part of this process; in itself it should not threaten the autonomy of professionals, but it should be seen as the process most likely to support the autonomy of patients.

If this process of decision-making is not initiated, and problems are left unresolved, stressful conflicts can occur, giving rise to intolerable interpersonal and interdisciplinary tensions that can be unhealthy and destructive to the team (Craig, 1996).

## Ethical skills and behaviour

Nurses should become advocates for a team approach to discussions around ethical decision-making, whereby no individual or professional perspective would have ultimate moral authority. All discussions should be focused on the needs of the patient. Furthermore, any fruitful discussion will rely on the cooperation of the health care team, and the capacity of each practitioner to act as a catalyst in the process of ethical decision-making (Tunna et al., 1993).

When a nurse says 'The doctor won't listen to me' that nurse needs to reflect on the situation and ask, 'How did I approach the doctor and the subject? Was I any of the following — aggressive, timid, articulate, knowledgeable of the facts, assertive, smiling, angry, confident — and could that have affected the doctor's response?' Aggressive behaviour from any member of the health care team will interfere with finding creative solutions.

Nurses need to be able to articulate their feelings and values openly and appropriately, and be able to empathise with other perspectives. Nurses need to listen to the opinions of colleagues, be nonjudgmental, deal with conflict constructively, and give and receive feedback without being defensive. If nurses wish truly to promote resolution of ethical problems they will need to be able to act as change agents and educators. Personal characteristics that will enhance the effectiveness of these skills include patience, honesty, trust, courage, understanding and empathy. Although many nurses already demonstrate these skills and characteristics, it needs to be acknowledged that, in practice, when it comes to dealing with common ethical problems, the skills and characteristics are not always being utilised.

If nurses continue to fail to distinguish between ethical dilemmas and ethical problems and put them both into the too-hard basket, both types of challenges will continue to be the major source of conflict within the health care team. Furthermore, they will continue to contribute to the high levels of stress that health care professionals already experience. However, if ethical dilemmas and problems are distinguished and recognised for what they are, then most of these ethical difficulties can, and should, be resolved.

## A SYSTEMATIC ETHICAL APPROACH

It is always helpful to use a conceptual approach to solving problems. Many decision-making or problem-solving models can be found in the nursing literature. For this text the SPIRAL model of decision-making (see Table 10.1) will be used.

A hypothetical case study will be presented to describe the process that nurses can use to achieve a practical solution to a common ethical problem.

**Table 10.1 SPIRAL model for decision-making**

| 1. | **SPECIFY** | Specify the problem and facts of the case |
|----|-------------|---------------------------------------------|
| 2. | **PRINCIPLES** | Identify the moral principles that bear on the case |
| 3. | **IDENTIFY** | Identify the options actually available |
| 4. | **REVIEW** | Review possible outcomes of action |
| 5. | **ACT** | Act effectively and with resolution |
| 6. | **LEARN** | Learn what you can by evaluating results |

(Reprinted from Thompson IE, Melia KM, 1995: *Nursing Ethics*, 3rd edn, by permission of the publisher, Churchill Livingstone)

## Case study

*Joe is a 65-year-old man diagnosed with metastatic colon cancer. He worked all his life as a schoolteacher until he retired 10 years ago. He lives with his wife and has three children.*

*Following Joe's initial operation the surgeon informed the wife and family that it had not been possible to remove all the cancer because it had spread to surrounding organs, in particular, the liver. Joe's pre-operative chest x-ray had also indicated the possibility of metastatic deposits. The surgeon informed the family that Joe's chances of long-term survival were very poor. The family asked the surgeon to conceal from their father the extent of the disease and the poor prognosis. The surgeon accepted their decision.*

*The oncology nursing staff met Joe when he arrived in the day centre for his first adjuvant chemotherapy treatment. The nursing staff had been informed by the oncology consultant that Joe knew he had cancer of the colon, but that he was not aware of the extent of his disease or of his poor prognosis.*

## 1. SPECIFY the problem and facts of the case

In order to identify clearly the problem or issues of any case, nurses need to have insight into their own personal and professional values. Furthermore, they need to acknowledge the potential differences between their values and the values of others who have an interest in the case. For example, the values of the patient, the family and other members of the health care team must also be considered.

The facts of the case presented are as follows:

- Joe is a patient who knows that he has cancer, but he has not been told the seriousness of his condition.

- His family want to protect him from receiving more bad news and have requested that this information be withheld from him.

- The surgeon, and subsequently the oncology consultant, have agreed to respect the family's wishes, and neither has explained to Joe the full extent of the disease or the poor chances of his long-term survival.

When Joe arrives in the day centre the nurses are likely to be alerted to this situation because of the potential problems it could create for ongoing communication, that is, effective communication between the family and the patient, the patient and the doctor, the patient and the nursing staff, and the family and the health care team.

One of the first responsibilities for the nurses administering Joe's chemotherapy is to ensure that he has a good understanding of his diagnosis, the treatment he is about to receive, and the potential side effects that could occur as a result of that treatment. Comprehensive patient education supports the concept of informed consent, and provides the nurse with an opportunity to establish a trusting relationship with Joe. The Australian Code of Ethics for nurses states that 'nurses respect the rights of persons to make informed choices in relation to their care'. Joe has a right to determine his own treatment, based on both the facts of his medical condition and his own personal values. Therefore, the nurses have some responsibility for ensuring that Joe is accurately informed about his condition, particularly if he asks. If nurses are forced to participate in a conspiracy of silence about Joe's prognosis, they are likely to experience a sense of discord about not fulfilling their responsibility. However, initially the nurses are likely to feel obliged to go along with the decision, mainly due to the possible consequences of going against the doctor's and the family's wishes.

In summary, the nurses are confronted with the problem of being placed in a compromising position between the patient, the family and the medical staff. The nurses may find themselves in disagreement with the doctor who has chosen to withhold certain information from Joe about his diagnosis and prognosis. As a result of that decision, the patient is being denied the opportunity to determine for himself what is in his best interests. The family are in disagreement with the nurses about the notion of beneficence (the promotion of benefits, including the balancing of benefits and harms) and non-maleficence (avoiding doing harm). While the family believe that to tell Joe will cause him more harm than good, the nursing staff may believe the opposite, that to give Joe the same information that everyone has will be of greater benefit to him than harm.

## 2. Identify the moral PRINCIPLES that bear on the case

Once the problem and facts of the case have been identified and clarified, the nurses need to identify the moral principles that will have relevance for this case. Nurses should use moral principles as starting points that give them direction and guidance; the principles do not in themselves provide answers to problems.

The principles considered relevant to this case will include the concept of **patient rights** and the responsibility of practitioners to respect those rights. The patient's right to know about his medical condition is generally derived from the principle of **autonomy** and respect for persons. If people are to be treated as persons with rights, that is the right to make informed choices and to exercise individual autonomy, then they cannot be denied the information necessary to enable them to make important life choices.

All of the interested parties will be concerned about doing what will benefit Joe most, and cause him least harm. These two concerns are derived from the principles of **non-maleficence** and **beneficence**.

Furthermore, the issue of **quality of life** should be raised. This will be particularly relevant if the chemotherapy that Joe is receiving not only offers him no chance of long-term survival, but also has the potential to produce side effects that will be distressing and have an impact on his quality of life.

It may be useful at this stage of identifying the problem, and the relevant moral principles, to reflect on any similar cases that have occurred in the past. To reflect on similar cases, and eventual outcomes of these (both positive and negative), will help guide the participants through the next step of decision-making, which is to identify possible actions.

## 3. IDENTIFY options actually available

To consider the various options when problem-solving an ethical issue, a number of different strategies can be used. These strategies are likely to include collaboration with members of the health care team and other relevant individuals and/or the coordination and facilitation of appropriate discussion forums where different perspectives can be expressed and heard. The nursing staff involved in these multidisciplinary discussions will need to give a reasoned account of their ethical position, and be able to offer some justification for the actions they are proposing. To do this, nurses will need to demonstrate an understanding of the key facts of the case, and the relevant moral principles that they have taken into consideration in reaching their position. The objective of these discussions should be aimed at reaching a decision which all participants can accept.

The practitioner who takes responsibility for this decision-making process will need to demonstrate the capacity to problem solve, and should possess the necessary interpersonal, groupwork and group leadership skills relevant to team-based decision-making and negotiation.

Therefore, a useful starting point when considering possible actions will be to seek explanation, and to reflect and consult with all of those involved. This requires that the nurses, the doctors and the relevant family members be willing to listen to one another's positions and perspectives in the interest of the best possible outcome for Joe. For example, the nurses need to make the doctor aware of the difficulties that they are experiencing as a result of not being able to talk honestly with Joe about his illness and possible outcomes. The nurses will want to gain a better understanding of why the family and the doctor chose to make the decision to withhold information from Joe in the first place. The family need to understand the full implications of their request. It will be necessary for health care professionals to mediate family discussions, and to provide ongoing counselling and support.

## 4. REVIEW possible outcomes of action

In order to be able to reach an agreement on the best action to take in this case, it will be necessary to discuss the potential outcomes of each proposed action.

If the decision is made to respect the principle of autonomy and tell Joe the truth about his condition, then it will be possible for the staff and family to offer their full support to Joe and assist him in coming to terms with his prognosis. Staff will be able to avoid feeling guilty about not telling the truth. The staff will then be in a better position to provide the necessary information to help Joe, and his family, consider their future options, and give them the opportunity to make the most out of what time Joe has left.

If the decision is made to continue to withhold certain information, then it is possible that Joe will gradually feel more anxious and suspicious about what is happening to him, particularly if people are avoiding the subject when they are around him. Furthermore, if Joe does feel alienated from those who care about him, he may become withdrawn and depressed, and react exactly the way the family feared he would if he had been told the bad news in the first instance. Staff will feel the burden of not telling the truth, and may find it increasingly difficult to answer any questions Joe asks. Joe will also be denied the opportunity to get his life affairs in order, and to do the important things he might want to before he dies.

Finally, consideration needs to be given to the possibility that the family and the doctor have made the right decision. If the family's intuition is right, and Joe does in fact prefer not to know the full extent of his condition, then to tell him may cause him further harm.

## 5. ACT effectively and with resolution

Once a decision has been made it will be important to act on it as soon as possible. A detailed description should be documented in the patient's history and should reflect all of the stages in the decision-making process, including a synopsis of the discussions that have taken place, and a clear plan of action. In addition, a process for ongoing review and reassessment should be clearly recorded.

It is worth noting that disagreements can occur at any stage of this process. They can arise over a disputation of the relevant facts, values or principles contributing to the case, or may be related to disagreement over what ought to be done, how it should be done, who should do it, how well it is actually done and whether the outcomes were successful.

In the event that any of the interested parties decline to be involved in the process, or an agreement cannot be reached, there are a number of other alternatives that nurses could consider. If the hospital has an ethics committee, nurses should know who their representative on that committee is, so that they can raise issues for discussion. There is also the Office of the Public Advocate that can be used in situations that might require the appointment of a patient advocate. Finally, if Joe requests the information from a member of the nursing staff, that person could choose to disregard the doctor's and family's wishes and tell Joe the truth (Johnstone, 1989).

## 6. LEARN what you can by evaluating results

As part of a continuous review of ethical practice, regular education sessions should be held to discuss ethical challenges that arise. Staff need to be given the opportunity to learn from experience and develop behaviours that will help prepare them for dealing with similar situations when they occur in the future. New policies or procedures will need to be developed or reviewed throughout this process.

Ethics rounds are just one way of approaching this review process constructively. Ethics rounds can deal with hypothetical cases, past case studies or current cases. It is important that these rounds are well organised and have a clear purpose. Ideally they are facilitated by an impartial person who has a sound knowledge of bioethical principles (Davis, 1982).

## Other problems

Joe's case as presented above can be resolved with careful consideration of all the issues. However, several new facts could be added to this case that would make it become a more complex and difficult dilemma. For example, Joe might be offered an experimental trial to test a new drug, without having a full understanding of the potential risks and benefits for him. Alternatively, Joe may be a practising Jehovah's Witness who has refused consent for blood transfusions, despite his treatment causing him symptomatic anaemia. He may have a psychiatric history of severe depressive illness and suicide attempts. Or Joe could unknowingly have been tested, and found to be positive, for the gene that is *thought* to be strongly associated with familial colon cancer. This raises another difficult ethical question: how should the family be advised?

Some of these more difficult problems may turn out to be resolvable. However, others will prove to result in an unresolvable clash of competing choices and/or values. These sorts of challenges will require a brave decision to be made under a veil of moral uncertainty, and there will need to be a preparedness by the decision-maker to live with the consequences of that decision, both good and bad.

## CONCLUSION

Situations involving patients with cancer will continue to provide ethical challenges for nurses providing care. Now, and even more so in the future, cancer nurses need to take more responsibility for dealing with those ethical challenges.

A famous nursing story tells of a patient who dies and finds himself in heaven. Uncertain of where he is he asks an angelic nurse, 'Nurse, where am I? Did I die?' The nurse replies, 'I think it would be best if you discussed that with the doctor.'

There is considerable opportunity for cancer nurses to facilitate and evaluate ethical decision-making processes, and in doing so they will contribute to the development of a dynamic and progressive professional ethic in cancer nursing.

## Acknowledgments

I would like to thank Kathy Swift and Sanchia Aranda for their valuable feedback to me while I was writing this chapter.

## References

Australian Nursing Council Inc. (1993): *Code of Ethics for Nurses in Australia*. Canberra: Australian Nursing Council Inc.

Craig YJ (1996): Patient : Medical ethics and mediation. *Journal of Medical Ethics* 22: 164–7.

Davis AJ (1982): Helping your staff address ethical dilemmas. *The Journal of Nursing Administration* February: 9–13.

Johnstone, M-J (1989): *Bioethics: A Nursing Perspective*. Sydney: W.B. Saunders/Balliere Tindall, p. 145.

Thompson IE, Melia KM, Boyd KM (1995): *Nursing Ethics*. New York: Churchill Livingstone.

Tunna K, Conner M (1993): You are your ethics. *The Canadian Nurse* May: 25–6.

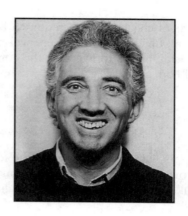

**TONY BUSH**
**Master of Primary Health Care, Bachelor of Applied Science,**
**Diploma of Applied Science, Registered Psychiatric Nurse, Registered Nurse,**
**Fellow of the Royal College of Nursing, Australia**
**Co-ordinator of a postgraduate course in cancer/palliative care nursing at**
**Royal Melbourne Institute of Technology (Bundoora Campus)**

Tony has worked in a number of countries and states in numerous clinical roles. He became aware that spirituality is a common feature of all persons regardless of background, but found it especially evident in people requiring oncological and palliative care. In more recent years, since completing postgraduate studies in palliative care, Tony has developed a model of spiritual care for use in a professional and a personal capacity. This appreciation of existential aspects has reaffirmed his belief that spiritual care really does have a place in the care of people with cancer and that any exploration of such matters will encourage the carer to undertake a personal journey of reflection, not just in their capacity as a nurse, but also in their role as a person.

Tony currently coordinates a postgraduate course in palliative care in which students are introduced to the topic of spirituality. This is a very popular aspect of the course and has resulted in Tony's examining various methods of facilitating students' exploration of spiritual concerns.

# Chapter 11

## *Spirituality — the essence of cancer care*

People who have been diagnosed with a cancer are often faced with a personal crisis, as they try to cope with a potentially life-threatening illness. This challenge to one's mortality is often recognised by cancer nurses as encompassing physical and psychosocial elements, but the spiritual component is often overlooked (Narayanasamy,1996; Taylor et al., 1994). This is indeed puzzling, given that holistic care is purported to include the areas of spirit and spirituality and that oncology nurses generally describe themselves as providers of holistic care (Taylor et al., 1994; Burkhardt, 1989). This caring in nursing usually includes empathy, sensitivity and compassion, qualities with which nurses are familiar and which are themselves very useful in the promotion of spiritual wellbeing (Diers, 1990). But is the provision of spiritual care really so important? Apparently it is, for even with cancer therapy improvements, the illness continues to be a major threat to life. Weisman and Worden (1976) describe the 100 days after diagnosis as a time of existential searching when patients become very concerned with the meaning of life, death and illness. A crucial time indeed and one in which the nurse is often privileged to accompany the patient struggling to cope with the diagnosis. In order to manage this major life change, patients employ spiritual coping strategies, often using nurses as resources for meeting spiritual needs (Sodestrom and Martinson, 1987).

But nurses generally do not facilitate patients' spirituality, even though cancer invariably creates such a need. The usual excuses proffered by nurses are that they believe spiritual matters to be outside their jurisdiction, mainly due to their lack of educational preparation, or they perceive anything spiritual to be the domain of a religious representative (Turner, 1996; Narayanasamy, 1993). This perception almost implies that spirituality refers only to patients and has no significance for nurses. Yet every person is a spiritual being with a spiritual dimension and many cancer nurses must have been faced with challenges to their own spiritual wellbeing when patients ask, 'Why me?' or 'What have I done to deserve this?' Such attempts to provide meaning within life are fundamental to everyone, although it usually requires a personal crisis for one to commence the search, and surely the diagnosis of a cancer is just such a time (Ersek and Ferrell, 1994). So whilst it appears that the role of spirituality has an integral part in oncology nursing, there still remains the question, what does the term 'spiritual' mean to nurses?

## WHAT IS SPIRITUALITY?

There are many definitions of the term spirituality and it is no wonder that nurses find the area so bewildering when it seems that no-one can agree on a single description.

The term 'spiritual' can be described as 'pertaining to the spirit of Man' and 'spirit' has been described as the 'breath of life which gives life to the physical organism' (Stoter, 1995:3). Other descriptions extend these concepts and describe the spiritual dimension as involving a search for meaning through a transcendent process, characterised by values important to oneself (Sherman, 1996). The principal theme is a search for meaning in life and for that meaning to be related to one's aspirations and responsibilities.

Many nurses have experienced the feelings of helplessness which arise when caring for cancer patients; not only do patients struggle to make sense of such seemingly vague concepts but nurses struggle too to find some personal meaning in the experience, to make some sense of it. Nurses unable to form these concepts into meaningful frameworks for themselves are very likely to not be able to assist patients searching for some meaning and are likely to give up any idea of helping patients to find answers to nonphysical concerns. This seems to be the case especially when caring for patients who are similar in age and background to the nurse, or who are particularly vulnerable, such as children. It is extremely difficult to make sense of these occasions by relying on one's own ability. Nurses will recall these occasions and how they themselves turned to an external force to guide them through this process of searching for meaning.

Whilst there are many descriptions of the term spirituality, an early definition by Renetzky (1979), still appears to be one of the more succinct and includes:

- the need to find meaning, purpose and fulfilment in life, suffering and death;

- the need for hope/will to live; and

- the need for belief and faith in self, others and God.

These components are developed and nurtured throughout one's life and are constantly reinforced by the shared experiences one has in interpersonal relationships. These experiences can obviously mean many things to many people, especially within a particular cultural context, and can provide a nurse with a unique opportunity to experience a variety of spiritual expressions. Sometimes these expressions reflect a person's religious beliefs, for example, observing a patient reading a specifically religious book such as the Bible. For patients with a religious preference, a search for meaning will be undertaken using that particular framework. Fry and Tan (1996) describe being religious as having a formal set of beliefs about God and using associated practices as a way to express one's spirituality on a regular basis. Another way of viewing spirituality can be by understanding the terms 'being' and 'doing'; the latter describes a patient's ability to undertake activities related to their role in society, whilst their being is the essence of who they are (Turner, 1996). This has a real relevance in cancer nursing, as it is common for a patient to be unable to maintain their usual role, focusing instead on an exploration of who they are in relation to their present circumstances.

The role of oncological therapies is of necessity an aggressive one, but to pay attention only to the treatments is to ignore the presence of the patient's being. In fact nurses themselves often overlook the fact that they also have a being requiring periodic examination as a means of making sense of their own life. By focusing on the technical care and ignoring the patients' and their own spiritual dimension, it is probable that nurses may evolve into nurses who happen to be people rather than people who happen to be nurses.

Some patients do not have a social support network, which is so important to a person coming to terms with a diagnosis of cancer (Sherman, 1996). Even if a patient is part of a family group, there are occasions when he/she chooses not to share concerns with individual family members; but there is still the need for the person to cope with the illness. As a means of coping, patients may rely more on the spiritual dimension and often turn to the nurse as a means of expressing their spiritual needs (Harrison, 1993). For many nurses this experience prompts them to reflect upon their own life and thus begin to uncover their own priorities and values. So begins a search for spiritual meaning.

## SEARCH FOR MEANING

To many patients, their families and indeed some health care professionals, the term cancer is synonymous with pain and suffering (Kahn and Steeves, 1995). This can be related to the disease itself, the treatments, or the potential for loss of life. It is also common for family members to experience their own suffering, in response to their loved one's trauma and this can be overlooked by health carers, as the attention is focused on the cancer patient. The patient's ability to find a personally relevant meaning in their suffering will often influence their ability to successfully adapt to the cancer (Ersek and Ferrell, 1994). For some nurses the whole issue of pain and suffering may be seen as belonging only to the physical domain and thus requiring only a physical therapy. The experience of suffering, however, affects not just the body but the whole person and any nursing intervention ought to reflect this distress as holistically as is possible (Kahn and Steeves, 1995). It might be easier said than done, however, when the nurse is faced with a patient suffering pain and experiencing a profound change to their quality of life. Questions such as, 'What have I done to deserve this?' are often asked by patients and are rarely able to be answered by their caregivers. Even though cancer nurses generally are quite knowledgeable about the clinical reasons for suffering, it is still not an easy topic to address. The very presence of suffering can be a challenge to a patient's mortality and can act as a reminder to the nurse that their life is also finite. In these situations it is not uncommon for the nurse to avoid discussion about the patient's meaning of suffering and to pay more attention to the actual clinical manifestations (Kahn and Steeves, 1995).

For some patients the illness is viewed as a punishment from God, or the result of personal health care practices; for example, it is common for a lung cancer sufferer to blame himself for the disease as a result of his smoking habit. Other patients perceive the disease to be bad luck, or 'just one of those things'. Whichever path the patient chooses, there is still a requirement for them to adjust to their new role, to identify what is really important to them and to be realistic about the possible outcomes of the disease (Narayanasamy, 1996). Since cancer has implications of suffering, the patient will rely not just on the available technologies, but will also commence a journey of introspection in the hope of being able to transcend their present situation. As the patient begins to explore the meaning of cancer pain, it's possible the nurse may identify three distinct meanings:

- immediate causes, when the patient expresses the belief that 'the pain means I'm really sick and am going to die';

- immediate effects of the pain, as evidenced by loss of role and independence, by helplessness and impact on family; and

- ultimate causes, such as the belief that, 'It's God's will', which can be associated with a spiritual distress.

Nurses usually see themselves as healers of pain. When faced with a patient who accepts pain as something to be endured, nurses may have to find a new role for themselves; they may have to rethink their own values. This can instigate the nurses' own search for meaning (Ersek and Ferrell, 1994).

Cancer nurses have a very special relationship with their patients and usually believe they can share in the patients' experiences by being empathetic and becoming involved in the illness experiences of their patients and the patients' families (Cohen, 1995). This 'being there' provides the nurse with a genuine connection to the patient and often encourages the nurse to decide what is truly important to them, not just in the work situation but within their personal life as well. As a result, nurses working with cancer patients are often able to find genuine meaning in their work and personal lives and may exhibit feelings of fulfilment and self-worth; by realising such meaning for themselves, nurses are able to intervene more appropriately with patients and families (Cohen, 1995).

A useful way to facilitate the patient's search for meaning is to suggest examining their lives from the earliest memory and to identify those events which have the greatest personal significance. By connecting past events and people to the present circumstances, the patient may begin to realise what is important to them in the future. Such a search usually leads to a re-evaluation of priorities and the realisation that one can rise above present circumstances (Birch, 1990). The reward for the nurse is to find the patient formulating their own meaning within their own context.

There are no instant answers to a search for meaning, but the personal rewards for both patient and nurse can be long lasting, and so the quest can be of value simply because it has begun.

*Helen was a 33-year-old mother of three, with cancer of the cervix and widespread metastases; her life expectancy was approximately 3–4 weeks. Her physical, social and emotional concerns were numerous, but she always had a smile and a cheerful greeting for the nurse. When asked how she managed in the presence of so many problems, she replied that she had a great family and a loving God — 'What more could a person want?' she would ask. As a result of repeated contacts with Helen, one of the nurses began to question aspects of her own life and commenced a re-evaluation of her own priorities: in fact she began her own search for meaning.*

Perhaps Nietzche best encapsulated this search, when he wrote, 'He who has a why to live can bear with almost any how' ( Frankl, 1964:vii).

## THE WILL TO LIVE

Hope provides spiritual sustenance for all patients, but is especially important for those people with a diagnosis of cancer (Ballard et al., 1997). It is one of the principal elements in making sense of a patient's search for meaning and provides a will to live and a sense of wellbeing and prevents the anguish of despair (Ross, 1995; O'Connor et al., 1990). Hope is so integral to a person's life that its loss can lead to premature death, for when a person loses control over life events, the effects of helplessness and hopelessness can result in 'passive suicide' (Ross, 1995, 1993; Renetzky, 1979).

Perhaps no-one is more aware of the need for hope than the patient with cancer. The hope that the diagnosis is wrong gives way to the hope that the treatment will be successful or that the symptoms will not be too disfiguring or painful. It appears, then, that there is more than one kind of hope. First there is the hope for recovery. When a cure is no longer evident, then a philosophical/theological hope transcends the process of dying (Rumbold, 1986). Cancer nurses will no doubt have witnessed such events on numerous occasions, but how can one describe such a nebulous topic as hope? In a broad sense hope refers to future expectations or wishes, but 'in medical usage the word seems to be limited implicitly to hope for recovery or survival' (Rumbold, 1986:59). Without hope, the patient begins to lose control over life, leading to feelings of helplessness. Such a state has been attributed not only to the disease, but also to prolonged inactivity, social isolation, a feeling of abandonment and, perhaps not surprisingly, uncertainties regarding one's spiritual, or, religious beliefs (Urden et al., 1992). All of these factors are commonly seen in cancer patients, particularly during the first few months of diagnosis and treatments, and are sometimes expressed as, 'What's the point?' or 'Why bother?' As the role of hope appears to be so crucial to a person's physical, psychosocial and spiritual wellbeing, how does one begin to maintain and promote it?

Having recognised the concept, the nurse can adopt the role of listener, by clarifying and reflecting, by supporting and by offering appropriate information when required (Rumbold, 1986). The role of reflection is particularly useful in working through the attendant emotions associated with the diagnosis, which need to be addressed before any other issues (Rumbold, 1986). The provision of any support should be grounded in a realistic context and comments such as, 'Don't worry, I'm sure it will be all right' do not reassure patients. Rather, such comments usually indicate that the caregiver is probably uncomfortable with the possibility of suffering and death. As a consequence, the patient may avoid sharing any personal concerns in future (Stoter, 1995). In order to nurture hope, the nurse must acknowledge the helping relationship as a two-way process, that patient and nurse will both receive any benefits from the exchange. '. . . nurses . . . play a key role in fostering hope in patients with cancer and their families . . . ' (Ballard et al., 1997:904).

*Kim was a 30-year-old woman with relapsed acute leukaemia. She disliked all the necessary attention related to her treatment and often appeared to be quite oblivious to the circumstances surrounding it. She had a very strong will to live, but her hope was implicitly tied in to her feigned ignorance of the seriousness of her illness; she maintained that 'this thing is not going to dominate my life'. Since she was doing so well it was probably not the time to remind her of possible relapse rates, but rather to support her in her desire to get well, and to be there for her, should she wish to raise any other concerns.*

# NEED FOR FAITH

A person's faith in themself and in God is often maintained by the love they receive from those around them. The need for love and worthwhile relationships is common to all people, and takes on a special emphasis during critical illness (Narayanasamy, 1996). For patients with a religious faith, it is important that they seek their God's love within this faith. However, there are many people who describe themselves as unbelievers and they seek their love through their relationships with family and friends. It does appear, though, that a person's spiritual wellbeing is enhanced if they have a formal belief in God (Renetzky, 1979). Within this belief, there also exists a sense of meaning, which can help to sustain a person through their illness.

For some patients the receipt of love comes from the nurse, in the way the nurse cares and ministers to the patient's needs (Harrington, 1995). Most nurses have found themselves providing unconditional compassion to a patient and have found it to be reciprocated, resulting in the nurse's own spiritual development being enriched. The unconditional nature of the giving will help give meaning and provide direction to the lives of both patient and nurse. When the focus of one's life is caring for others, then one can live the meaning of one's life (Millison and Dudley, 1990).

For patients coping with cancer, religious practices and spirituality are important because they reduce the anxiety associated with the illness and provide decreased levels of pain, anger and social isolation and higher levels of life satisfaction (Jenkins and Pargament, 1995). It appears that cancer nurses share similar ways of coping with job-related stress — they draw upon their religious faith and the support of their friends and family (Wilkinson, 1994). For those without any structured beliefs, meditation, in whatever fashion, has been found useful (Wilkinson, 1994).

One element is common to all cancer patients and that is the need for a social network from which the patient can draw the compassion and love so essential to survival; it often falls upon the nurses to provide these qualities in the absence of a network. Nurses should not be disheartened and think this is just one more task to do, as it is by loving that the caregiver promotes the patient's spiritual growth and this will help to create the conditions necessary for the carer's own growth (Peck, 1978).

*Jack was a 62-year-old man with cancer of the oesophagus. He lived alone, with no significant social network and professed no beliefs in God or any religious faith. His condition was such that he was going to require artificial feeding methods in order to maintain life. He confided in the nurse that he really didn't want this, as it meant his quality of life would be unbearable and 'anyway who would miss me?' Three days after making this treatment decision, Jack died; his primary nurse was with him and it was apparent that she was the only person filling his need for compassion. After his death the nurse was heard to remark, 'Jack's dying alone made me rethink my own position on the importance of relationships!'*

## SUGGESTIONS FOR SPIRITUAL CARE

It's probably fair to say that cancer nurses have many opportunities to provide spiritual care given that a diagnosis of cancer often initiates spiritual needs (Taylor et al., 1994). However there appears to be some confusion over the term 'spiritual care', largely due to nurses not understanding what is meant by the term spirituality (Taylor et al., 1994). Nurses who read this chapter may gain a clearer understanding of spirituality and a preparedness to facilitate a patient's spiritual needs. The skills required are somewhat different from those needed to implement any physical therapy and to some extent require more effort from the nurse. It is not always an easy task to undertake, but the benefits for the patient and the nurse are many; instead of a nurse just 'doing something' for the patient, the nurse can now 'be there' with that person. This state of 'being' is reflective of true caring and is a feature of job satisfaction for cancer nurses (Wilkinson, 1994).

Probably one of the more specific requirements for cancer nurses is to be aware of their own values, attitudes and beliefs and to be comfortable in the knowledge that these are often going to be at odds with those of the patients (Narayanasamy, 1996; Stoter, 1995).

*Elizabeth was a 55- year-old woman with metastatic breast cancer and a poor prognosis. She had a tendency to irritate nursing staff as a result of her frequent wish to be discharged during chemotherapy. She believed it was more important to spend time with her partner in her own home rather than remain in hospital. Her attitudes and values were at variance with the majority of the ward staff who saw it as their role to be more prescriptive in terms of what Elizabeth ought to be doing. One nurse, recognising Elizabeth's will to live combined with her search for meaning, was the only nurse comfortable in supporting Elizabeth's choice.*

This illustration highlights the need for any caregiver to have examined their own spirituality, to accept it and to be able to enter into a caring relationship through being willing to accept the patient on their terms (Narayanasamy, 1993). To be comfortable with the area of spiritual matters appears to be almost a prerequisite for anyone working in the area of oncology. When spirituality is integrated within a religious faith it appears that cancer nurses will cope much better with the stresses of their work (Wilkinson, 1994).

Genuineness and willingness to facilitate a patient's spiritual concerns are also required, but to be part of good caring, these need to be incorporated with competence. Many nurses can correctly claim that they already use such skills, as any caring in nursing usually includes the use of empathy, sensitivity and compassion (Diers, 1990). However, instead of believing these skills to be peculiar to nursing, try to realise that they are potential features of everyone, just as spirituality is. This perception will encourage nurses to believe that, though such features are important, they must be translated into practice to be considered effective. Many opportunities arise for the cancer nurse to help a patient in the search for meaning, even within the often frantic pace of an oncology ward. Those nurses who use occasions such as showering or changing IV flasks to offer the patient support are saying to the patient, 'You are important to me and even though I'm busy, I want to listen to your concerns'. Because the nurse is expressing a genuine concern, a feeling of trust will develop, which is essential to the creation of a suitable milieu for the expression of spiritual thoughts and feelings (Narayanasamy, 1996).

For many people communication skills mean talking to one another. To some extent this is true in spiritual care, but a more useful skill is the nurse being very comfortable with the use of silence. Patients often express themselves in a way which is designed not to give offence to their audience — the nurse. As a consequence the nurse has to listen actively, usually without interruptions, in order to hear what is being said and, often, what is not said. If it is culturally appropriate, eye contact can help maintain contact during these exchanges.

*Bob was a 44-year-old man with bowel cancer. He often appeared to be apprehensive but never quite managed to verbalise his concerns. One day he asked the nurse, 'Do you believe the treatment will work?' The nurse responded with 'What do you feel about it?' This allowed Bob a beginning and he spoke at some length about his concerns regarding the possibility of dying. The nurse said nothing during this time, but managed to convey her interest by maintaining periodic eye contact. In fact it transpired that Bob was experiencing a major spiritual crisis and was referred to a pastoral care worker. But it was the primary nurse who instigated it, and without her empathy, listening skills and working knowledge of spiritual care, this episode could have turned out very differently.*

During such times, it is advisable that both the nurse and the patient share the same meaning of the words used. There are times when nurses forget that the patient may be so fearful that any dialogue is incomprehensible, or the patient's age might mean contemporary words have little meaning. Always reply to the patient by summarising what the patient has said so that they have the opportunity to correct any misunderstanding (Stoter, 1995). Sometimes a patient may ask about the nurse's own spiritual beliefs. This appears to act as a reminder for the nurse to give thought to the spiritual dimension, which often results in spiritual growth for both patient and nurse (Narayanasamy, 1996).

*Jimmy was a single man in his late 60s with no next of kin and no friends. Most of his life had been spent as a prospector. He had lung cancer which was being treated palliatively. His main enjoyment was playing chess with the staff. During one of these games he asked the nurse if she believed in life after death. The nurse hesitated then affirmed she did and said why. Jimmy listened attentively and expressed his views of life, death, and dying, most of which were related to a relationship with Nature. This was the first time he had spoken in depth and both he and the nurse had many more such exchanges before he died. The nurse commented on how Jimmy's beliefs did not alter hers, but allowed her to rethink aspects of her life which previously she had ignored. By using her own religious faith to explore their spirituality, she was able to reflect the claim that this '. . . has also been identified as a factor which facilitates good communication between nurses and cancer patients' (Wilkinson, 1994:1083).*

Many nurses are familiar with the communication skills described in this chapter but have probably not thought about using them in the provision of spiritual care. When used in conjunction with the concepts of spirituality, they can enhance not just the patients' wellbeing, but also promote the wellbeing of nurses. One of the key roles for oncology nurses is being able to participate in the patient's experiences by forming relationships and 'being there' in all the phases of the patient's illness (Cohen, 1995). How much more satisfying then for the nurse to be able to incorporate the spiritual dimension within caring; not only does it provide the patient with a means of examining critical life issues, it also gives the opportunity for the nurse to experience greater job satisfaction, as well as personal satisfaction (Wilkinson, 1994; Birch, 1990).

## CONCLUSION

During the past decade there has evolved an appreciation of the role of spirituality and its practical application within the clinical domain. There is ample evidence to support the claim that meeting a cancer patient's spiritual needs can also diminish the severity of their symptoms, thus reducing the need for prescribed therapies. Not only patients but also cancer nurses can benefit from the provision of spiritual care. Providing spiritual care to the patient can lead to the exploration of the nurse's own spiritual needs in a meaningful way, which will provide support and direction in both personal and professional life.

Coming to terms with their own spirituality can be a key factor in maintaining cancer nurses throughout the many personal and professional crises faced in such a demanding clinical area; it can also assist in the prevention of burnout by providing nurses with ways in which meaning can be found in their work and life.

## References

Ballard A, Green T, McCaa A, Logsdeon C (1997): A comparison of the level of hope in patients with newly diagnosed and recurrent cancer. *Oncology Nursing Forum* 24 5: 899–904.

Birch C (1990): *On Purpose.* Sydney: New South Wales University Press Ltd.

Burkhardt MA (1989): Spirituality: An analysis of the concept. *Holistic Nursing Practice* 3 3: 69–77.

Cohen MZ (1995): The meaning of cancer and oncology nursing: Link to effective care. *Seminars in Oncology Nursing* 11 1: 59–67.

Diers D (1990): To Profess . . . To Be a Professional. In Lindemann C and McAthie M (eds): *Nursing Trends and Issues.* Springhouse, Pennsylvania: Springhouse.

Ersek M, Ferrell BR (1994): Providing relief from cancer pain by assisting in the search for meaning. *Journal of Palliative Care* 10 4: 15–22.

Frankl V (1964): *Man's Search for Meaning*. London: Hodder and Stoughton.

Fry A, Tan L (1996): The spiritual dimension: Its importance to the nursing care of older people. *Geriaction* 14 4: 14–17.

Harrington A (1995): Spiritual care: What does it mean to RNs? *Australian Journal of Advanced Nursing* 12 4: 5–14.

Harrison J (1993): Spirituality and nursing practice. *Journal of Clinical Nursing* 2: 211–217.

Jenkins RA, Pargament KI (1995): Religion and spirituality as resources for coping with cancer. *Journal of Psychosocial Oncology* 13 1–2: 51–74.

Kahn DL, Steeves RH (1995): The significance of suffering in cancer care. *Seminars in Oncology Nursing* 11 1: 9–16.

Millison M, Dudley J (1990): The importance of spirituality in hospice work: A study of hospice professionals. *Hospice Journal* 6 3: 63–78.

Narayanasamy A (1996): Spiritual care of chronically ill patients. *British Journal of Nursing* 5 7: 411–416.

Narayanasamy A (1993): Nurses' awareness and educational preparation in meeting their patients' spiritual needs. *Nurse Education Today* 13: 196–201.

O'Connor AP, Wicker CA, Germino BB (1990): Understanding the cancer patient's search for meaning. *Cancer Nursing* 13: 167–175.

Peck S (1978): *The Road Less Travelled : A New Psychology of Love, Traditional Values and Spiritual Love*. London: Arrow Books.

Renetzky L (1979): The Fourth Dimension: Applications to the Social Services. In: Moberg DO (ed.): *Spiritual Well-being: Sociological Perspectives*. Washington: University Press of America, pp. 215–254.

Ross LA (1993): Spiritual aspects of nursing. *Journal of Advanced Nursing* 19: 439–447.

Ross LA (1995): The spiritual dimension: Its importance to patients' health, well-being and quality of life and its implications for nursing practice. *International Journal of Nursing Studies* 32 5: 457–468.

Rumbold BD (1986): *Hopelessness and Hope: Pastoral Care in Terminal Illness*. London: SCM Press Ltd.

Sherman DW (1996): Nurses' willingness to care for AIDS patients and spirituality, social support, and death anxiety. *IMAGE: Journal of Nursing Scholarship* 28 3: 205–213.

Sodestrom KE, Martinson IA (1987): Patients' spiritual coping strategies: A study of nurse and patient perspectives. *Oncological Nursing Forum* 14 2: 41–46.

Stoter D (1995): *Spiritual Aspects of Health Care*. Times Mirror International Publishers Ltd.

Taylor EJ, Highfield M, Amenta M (1994): Attitudes and beliefs regarding spiritual care: A survey of cancer nurses. *Cancer Nursing* 17 6: 479–487.

Turner P (1996): Caring more, doing less. *Nursing Times* 21 August, 92 34.

Urden LD, Davis JK, Thalan LA (1992): *Essentials of Critical Care Nursing*. St Louis: CV Mosby.

Weisman AD, Worden JW (1976): The existential plight in cancer: Significance of the first 100 days. *International Journal of Psychiatry Medicine* 7: 1–15.

Wilkinson SM (1994): Stress in cancer nursing: Does it really exist? *Journal of Advanced Nursing* 20: 1079–1084.

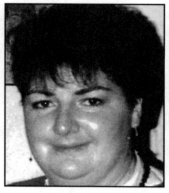

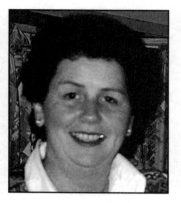

Karen Glaetzer

Alison Mcleod

## KAREN GLAETZER
Registered Nurse, Oncology Certificate, Bachelor of Nursing
Clinical Nurse Consultant Palliative Care Outreach,
Repatriation General Hospital/Southern Community Hospice Program,
Adelaide, South Australia

Karen Glaetzer completed her general training at the Repatriation General Hospital, Daw Park, in Adelaide, in 1982. In 1984 she undertook the Post Basic Oncological Nursing Course at Peter MacCallum Cancer Institute, Melbourne. In 1988, on returning to South Australia, Karen assisted in establishing Daw House Hospice. In 1989 she pioneered the Palliative Care Liaison role with the Repatriation General Hospital. While working in this position Karen has been involved in the development and coordination of the Intensive Course in Palliative Care Nursing offered by The Flinders University of South Australia/International Institute of Hospice Studies. She also provides a consultancy service to the Ashford Cancer Centre. In 1997 she was involved in palliative care courses in Thailand, Vietnam, The Philippines and New Zealand.

## ALISON McLEOD
Registered Comprehensive Nurse, Oncology Certificate,
Bachelor of Business (Human Resource Management)
Member of the Royal College of Nursing, Australia
Clinical Nurse Consultant, Daw House Hospice, Adelaide, South Australia

Alison McLeod completed her Registered Comprehensive Nursing Education at Auckland Technical Institute, New Zealand, in 1980. She undertook the Post Basic Oncological Nursing Certificate at Peter MacCallum Cancer Institute, Melbourne, in 1985. After moving to Adelaide, Alison was Clinical Nurse Consultant at the Philip Kennedy Centre Hospice before accepting a position at Daw House Hospice. As the Inpatient Clinical Nurse Consultant Alison has been involved in the development and coordination of the Intensive Course in Palliative Care Nursing offered by The Flinders University of South Australia/International Institute of Hospice Studies. Alison has travelled to Hong Kong, China, Fiji and New Zealand to provide palliative care courses to multidisciplinary teams.

# Chapter 12

## *Palliative care — an integrated part of cancer care*

## INTRODUCTION

Hospice care, palliative care and terminal care are all terms used to describe interventions that provide comfort and symptom control to those with terminal illnesses.

The word 'hospice' is derived from the Latin word 'hospes' meaning host or guest. Hospices were known to be in existence in the Middle Ages and were places where travellers and pilgrims were cared for.

'Palliative' arises from the Latin root pallus, to mask, and refers to the alleviation of symptoms.

The word 'terminal' is a little more difficult to define as it can be used in the context of someone having a terminal illness but who may live for some years. It is also used by nurses working in palliative care to describe the final hours or days. You will hear nurses say that someone who has been ill for some time is now 'terminal'.

All of these terms are to some degree interchangeable and Australia has acknowledged both hospice and palliative care by titling its national body the 'Australian Association of Hospice and Palliative Care'.

This Association defines palliative care (AAHPC, 1994) as:
> . . . a concept of care which provides coordinated medical nursing and allied services for people who are terminally ill, delivered where possible in the environment of the person's choice and which provides physical, psychological, emotional and spiritual support for patients, families and friends. The provision of

hospice and palliative care services includes grief and bereave-ment support for the family and other carers during the life of the patient and continuing after death.

Why is palliative care a new specialty? Why is it only now that we have palliative care for the dying? It is not as if dying is new.

Doyle (1993) discusses how, at one time, all care of those with cancer was palliative, as there were no treatments. The same could be said of many other diseases. As medical science discovered surgical, pharmacological and medical cures, the emphasis of care became treatment. In both medicine and nursing it could be said that we lost sight of the need to provide comfort care in the midst of an environment focused on cure.

With encouragement by governments for members of society to take more responsibility for their own health, and an increasing demand by people to exercise choice, nursing practice is being forced to change, and service delivery is being expected to meet the needs of patients rather than the needs of professional organisations such as hospitals.

If we consider what has impacted on the delivery of good palliative care nursing, two issues emerge:

1.  The fear of death and the difficulty both the community and health care professionals have had in accepting that there is no cure for some illnesses, and that death is inevitable.

2.  The culture of nursing and the organisation within which nurses work, whether that be within an inpatient facility or in the community.

In this chapter, with the use of case studies, we will demonstrate how the integration of palliative care and acute care assists both health care professionals and patients to overcome their fear of the process of death.

We will identify changes that need to be made in attitudes and beliefs of nurses, and demonstrate that those wishing to provide good palliative care need to build on their knowledge and skills and to examine why they practise the way they do.

## WHEN DEATH IS INEVITABLE

It has been estimated that 90 per cent of patients referred for palliative care have a diagnosis of cancer. Historically, palliative care has been viewed as beginning when all attempts at cure have been exhausted.

More recently, palliative care has been viewed as a discipline of care and support which is able to complement cancer treatment and extend into the bereavement phase. Using this model, the distress for the patient is reduced and the palliative care team is seen as a service which is responsive to needs as the patient and family perceive them. As treatment options become fewer, palliative care involvement increases. This is a gradual process called 'parallel care' rather than an abrupt 'handing over', and highlights the advantage of hospital-based teams which are also able to access community resources (Maddocks, 1996). Initial palliative care contact may be offered in an outpatient clinic. As the disease progresses, a home visit by a palliative care team member is much more compatible with the needs of the patient. Here, the patient is able to be viewed as an integral part of a larger unit which is the network of family and friends. Home consultations tend to be more relaxed and comprehensive. Patients are able to be reassured that they are not being abandoned, that the major change has been the site of care rather than a change of care provider.

So how do we encourage early involvement of palliative care services? This question needs to be tackled from both a professional and a public perspective.

First, we need to accept that many cancers are not curable and treatment from the outset is aimed at palliation (Scott, 1979). Secondly, we need to acknowledge the valuable contribution which palliative care services make, complementing the services offered by oncology services.

What is required is a change of attitude. Referral to palliative care services can be seen as having negative connotations, being thought of as surrendering, as giving up hope. Palliative care services themselves need to carry some of the responsibility for this attitude, as referrals were declined in the past if there was any hint that the patient may live too long. Palliative care professionals have now accepted the difficulties in predicting prognosis and embraced the importance of early involvement. Now we need to promote this philosophy amongst other medical specialties such as cardiology, respirology and, most importantly, oncology. In some circumstances it may be quite appropriate for oncology services to remain the major care provider, but we need to remember that medical oncology focuses on treating the disease, while palliative care is based on treating symptoms which the disease causes. The ideal situation, therefore, is a partnership which offers patients a full range of options.

## CHANGING THE FOCUS

The modern hospice movement, being a relatively new concept of care, has opened a number of opportunities for providers to review and question historic health care practices. This section of the chapter will examine the barriers to providing good palliative care in nursing.

Good palliative care nursing is an essential component of nursing the person with cancer and other terminal illnesses but there are a number of barriers to good palliative care nursing entrenched in the culture of modern health institutions and, more significantly, in the tradition of nursing. These barriers result in the continuation of routine procedures which impinge on valuable time that could be better spent meeting needs identified by the patient. Measuring urine, doing daily weights and recording vital signs are examples of traditional nursing practice which, at times, can be uncomfortable and disruptive for ill patients. These routines prevent comfort care, especially when they are undertaken in an acute setting or when the patient has been receiving, and indeed expects to continue receiving, treatment with a view to cure.

Effective palliative care is primarily about providing comfort care. The Oxford Dictionary (1991) defines comfort as
> consolation, relief of affliction, a state of physical wellbeing,
> things that make life easy or pleasant.

Comfort is a subjective state and in palliative care health professionals rely on patients and carers to say what will relieve discomfort, what will make life easy and pleasant.

Let us for a moment consider what a culture is. It could be defined as 'the way things are done around here' (Shafritz and Ott, 1996:35). Cultures are made up of traditions, mores, values, unwritten rules, policies and procedures, and it is these that contribute to nurses having difficulty transferring their focus of care from cure to comfort, from institution and nursing focus to patient focus.

Delivering effective palliative care in an acute oncological setting is most difficult as it requires the nursing team to make a major shift in the way they assess, plan and deliver care. In an acute setting the focus is on what the patient needs to be cured. When palliative care patients are assessed the emphasis is placed on what the patient requests to maintain a quality of life. Palliative care aims to be proactive in the management of symptoms, for example, providing good pain control, preventing constipation and alleviating anxiety, while aiming to reduce the number of interventions. Palliative care should allow the natural process of dying to occur, while maintaining maximum comfort.

The key to changing the nurses' focus is achieved by placing the patient's comfort first and this can sometimes cause a number of dilemmas.

## Changing routine management

*A patient with terminal cancer is admitted to the unit for symptom control. The patient is also a diabetic controlled with diet and tablets. On admission the patient is put on the same regime that she has been on at home which includes twice daily blood sugar readings. A few days after admission it becomes apparent that the patient is deteriorating and will not go home again. The patient is anorexic and cannot tolerate a full diabetic diet. What are the dilemmas?*

- *Should the nurse subject the patient to finger pricks twice daily?*

- *Should the diet of a dying person be restricted?*

- *Is the patient anxious that his/her diabetic regime remains the same?*

- *As the person nears death, if hypoglycaemia or hyperglycaemia occurs, should it be treated?*

- *Are the family anxious about the patient not eating?*

In palliative care it may well be appropriate to:

- cease blood sugar readings as they are uncomfortable

- allow the patient to eat and drink whatever is wanted as it is often only a small amount anyway

- treat symptoms of hypoglycaemia or hyperglycaemia only if they occur

- ensure that the patient and the family are included in all decision making

It is difficult to change the focus from the rigid management of patients with diet- and tablet-controlled diabetes to a more flexible approach.

In nursing, many of our practices have evolved from an emphasis on what we believed was important and necessary at that time. We now have practices firmly implanted in our clinical environment that are not conducive to the provision of good palliative care.

## Ritual as practice

*Recently a palliative care nurse was asked to help out in an acute medical ward on a Sunday morning. Following morning handover she was passed a weigh seat and was asked to weigh all the patients on the south side of the unit. The nurse questioned whether it was necessary to ask all 16 patients to leave their warm beds on a Sunday morning, suggesting that not all needed weighing. She was told that all patients on the north side of the ward were weighed on Saturday and the rest on Sunday, . . . 'because we always do'.*

This is an example of a nursing practice that has become entrenched in the ward culture. It subjects patients to unnecessary interventions and serves little useful purpose, particularly for patients who have cancer, are weak and are obviously losing weight. How could this time be utilised better?

It is so easy for us to continue on with 'the routine', leading to inappropriate interventions without consciously acknowledging that the focus of care has altered from cure to comfort.

## Challenging routine nursing practice

*A palliative care nurse consultant was asked to visit an acute medical ward where the nurses were caring for a patient dying of cancer. The patient had oozing, painful blisters on his hands and feet. The blisters were being dressed twice daily. Prior to dressings additional pain relief was being given. The problem for the nurses was that the family were concerned that the extra analgesic made their father drowsy and he could not interact with them as they wished. The nurses wanted to know what analgesia and what amount would best meet the needs of the patient. The nurses' focus was right. They wanted the patient to have comfort and the family to have quality time. The palliative nursing consultant simply asked, 'Why are you doing the dressings?'*

*The blisters were left open and the man's hands and feet were placed on absorbent towels so there was no need to continue with dressings.*

Sometimes we continue nursing practices simply because we always have. For patients receiving palliative care nurses must think laterally, step away from routine practice, and recognise that if a practice is not going to achieve comfort for the patient, then it should be discarded. In relation to wounds, if there is no hope or need for the wound to heal, the focus should be changed to comfort care. The difficulty is knowing when to make the switch from cure to comfort. Many cancer patients are already receiving treatment that is palliative, even though there is an expectation that their life will have quantity and quality. When should the emphasis of care change?

## ASSESSMENT

The key to providing effective palliative care is in the careful, patient-focused assessment of the needs of the person with cancer, together with consideration for patients, family and friends. Treatment decisions should be guided by the establishment of mutual goals. When identifying patient problems and needs it is important that the person being cared for and the carers be consulted. Assessment should be made from their perspective.

Dunlop (1989), when studying the degree of distress caused by symptoms, found that many symptoms rated high in distress by patients were rated low by health professionals, and vice versa. This can result in nurses wanting to implement interventions which are not welcomed because they are not a priority for the patient. The patient's concerns must be heard.

# What is good nursing and what is bad nursing?

*A man was admitted to a hospice unit with dyspnoea. He had been living at home alone, becoming increasingly unkempt due to his inability t o mobilise without experiencing extreme shortness of breath. On admission, he was unshaven and unwashed and his mouth and tongue were thickly coated with thrush and drying sputum. A priority for nurses was to intervene with vigorous mouth care and provide simple hygiene. The man resisted and became quite angry about this, as his major concern was the fact that he felt he was going to suffocate any minute. It was 24 hours later, and only after his dyspnoea was controlled, that he would accept mouth care and hygiene*

Nurses often find it difficult to stand back because nursing culture has indoctrinated them with the belief that nonintervention results in bad nursing.

Using a palliative approach nurses need to:

- address the patient's concerns first

- control physical symptoms in line with the patient's priority

- be aware of the impact on the patient of emotional/spiritual/social distress

- accept that not all symptoms can be alleviated, thereby avoiding inappropriate optimism

- be prepared to be technical and scientific or humble and homespun in controlling symptoms

- be prepared to explain what, why, when and how in every detail

Palliative care gives nurses the opportunity to examine every care they give and ask, 'Why am I doing this?' If the answer is 'because that is what we have always done', or 'that is what I learned to do in my training', or 'because that is what I think should be done', then the next question to be asked is 'Is this intervention going to alleviate discomfort for this patient, and does this patient want me to do this?'

## NURSING AND THE TIME FACTOR

Health care has always been a victim of the time factor. Nurses frequently claim that we do not have sufficient time to spend with our patients; so we must ensure that we make the best use of the time we do have.

We need to adopt the same message we give our patients, we must make whatever time is available quality time. We may not have the time available to sit and talk to patients, but we can incorporate listening and talking into all patient contact time. When assisting patients with their hygiene needs, we can use the time to allow them to vent their fears and discuss any issues of concern. We can ensure that every interaction is a worthwhile experience.

# PUBLIC PERCEPTIONS

As has been mentioned already, members of society, in recent times, have tended to take more responsibility for their own health. The public now are more inclined to question interventions when in the past they accepted whatever was offered. Some will decide from the outset that they do not want any life-prolonging treatments. All of us, as members of society and particularly as nurses, need to be able to accept the individual's right to choose, even though this may contradict our beliefs.

It is unreasonable to expect everyone to reach the same level of acceptance. The more discussion on this subject that takes place, the closer we come to adopting a more positive view from which society as a whole will benefit. When we as nurses offer patients a range of options for treating a life-threatening illness, we have an obligation to include palliative care. This alone will enhance the public's perception of palliative care.

## A case study approach to integrated care

*Susan was 32 years old when she presented to her general practitioner with unspecific symptoms of lethargy, tiredness and abdominal discomfort. The symptoms had been present for some weeks, but initially she felt they were related to the added stress of moving house. On examination, her general practitioner detected hepatomegaly and arranged further investigations. She was diagnosed with liver metastases. She was referred to an oncologist who ordered further investigations, which failed to detect a primary site. This limited the treatment options and proved to be a source of ongoing anxiety for Susan, as she had difficulty understanding why the source of the cancer could not be found.*

*Susan had two sons, Sam aged 13 and David aged 5. She had been separated from their father, Roger, for two years and he now lived interstate. When told of Susan's diagnosis, he returned and proved to be her major support. He also accepted ongoing responsibility for the children.*

*Susan was offered a course of continuous 5-fluorouracil in an attempt to control the rapidly progressing disease. An infusaport was inserted so that she could be an outpatient. The disease progressed but Susan remained reluctant to cease what she viewed as her only hope of a cure. The palliative care team was asked to make contact, which she accepted. This first contact was in a clinic conducted at the cancer centre where she was receiving treatment. This allowed the palliative care team involvement to be seen as an extension of the services offered by the centre.*

*At this consultation her main symptoms were assessed by the health care team to be:*

- *increasing ascites*
- *leg oedema presumably due to hypoalbumanaemia*
- *liver tenderness*
- *anorexia and vomiting due to squashed stomach syndrome*
- *dry mouth with evidence of oral thrush.*

*As is common practice in palliative care, Susan was encouraged to rate her symptoms from her perspective. She identified insomnia as her highest priority, due to discomfort from increasing ascites. At this initial contact six litres of fluid was drained via a jelco in the left iliac fossa. She was commenced on:*

- *slow-release morphine 20 mg bd*
- *immediate-release morphine 10 mg 2 hourly prn*
- *dexamethasone 4 mg mane to reduce peri-tumour oedema*
- *metoclopramide 10 mg ac to increase gastric emptying*
- *dothiapen 25 mg nocte to improve sleep*
- *ranitidine 150 mg bd*
- *nilstat 1 ml qid.*

*The next day she phoned to say she had had her best night's sleep for weeks. She had also been delaying a short holiday, but decided now the time was right. Plans were made for her to attend the hospital in the holiday town if paracentesis was required.*

*Initial consultation continued at the cancer centre on a weekly basis. This enabled review of her pain management and drainage of her ascites. As her condition deteriorated, home visits by the same team were initiated. Leg oedema became an increasing problem and complementary therapy services were organised via the palliative care team. A social worker made contact with Roger and the children.*
*Eventually, chemotherapy was ceased when the side effects, mainly*

*stomatitis, became intolerable. Susan was extremely disappointed and eager to pursue other avenues, but she was also beginning to accept the seriousness of her situation. Her condition deteriorated steadily over the next few weeks and when home care became impossible she was admitted to the private hospital linked to the cancer centre where she died peacefully*

*24 hours later. Bereavement care was provided by the palliative care service.*

By integrating care, a support system eventuated that enabled Susan to maintain links with oncology services who offered her hope and palliative care services who assisted her and her family to face reality.

## CONCLUSION

In this chapter a model of care has been demonstrated that recognises palliative care as a positive step in the management of patients with advanced cancer. By combining the knowledge and skills of all specialities, by challenging nurses' attitudes and beliefs about the care they deliver and by recognising the need to change many of the traditions, rituals, mores, policies and procedures that have developed within nursing cultures over the decades, we can help patients to look forward to a greater quality of life.

Hospital-based palliative care services allow ongoing involvement by the same team from initial contact through to the bereavement phase. Using this model the public and professional perspective of palliative care services will be enhanced. The focus moves from being portrayed as 'the death squad' to a team of professionals providing high-quality supportive care.

The model of care used in the provision of palliative care, if adopted in other health care settings, would challenge nurses to review their attitudes and beliefs and dispense with outdated traditions. This would in turn enhance nursing practice.

## References

Australian Association for Hospice and Palliative Care (AAHPC) Inc. (1994): *Standards for Hospice Palliative Care Provision*. March.

*The Concise Oxford Dictionary of Current English* (1991): Oxford: Clarendon Press.

Doyle D (1993): *Oxford Textbook of Palliative Medicine*. Oxford: Oxford University Press. Dunlop GM (1989): A study of the relative frequency and importance of gastrointestinal symptoms, and weakness in patients with far advanced cancer: Student paper. *Palliative Medicine* 4: 37–43.

Maddocks I (1996): *Palliative Care. A Guide for General Practitioners*. (5th edn). Daw Park, South Australia: Southern Hospice Foundation.

Scott RB (1979): *Cancer the Facts*. Oxford: Oxford University Press.

Shafritz Jay M, Ott J Steven (1996): *Defining Organisational Culture*. California USA: Wadsworth Publishing Co., p. 35

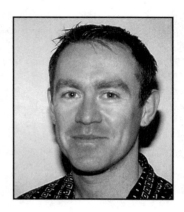

**CAMERON A. SINCLAIR**
**Registered Nurse, Bachelor of Science, Bachelor of Nursing (Honours)**

After completing his science degree in 1989, Cameron returned to university in 1992 to study nursing, and graduated with honours. Upon obtaining his nurse registration he worked in an oncology/haematology unit which inspired his honours study. His project, titled 'How nurses interact with significant others when an oncology patient dies', considered interactions that occurred between nurses and the significant others of oncology clients. The aim of the study was to identify supportive strategies oncology nurses employed with significant others at and around the time of a client's death.

Cameron currently works in an Infectious Diseases and HIV/AIDS unit in which people suffering neoplastic diseases are a substantial proportion of his client group. Cameron maintains an interest in education by teaching and assessing tertiary students in areas of health and first aid.

# Chapter 13

## *Caregiver support*

## INTRODUCTION

A diagnosis of cancer can throw anyone into a state of chaos and turmoil. For many it is often paramount to a death sentence. Issues surrounding mortality, grief and loss are encountered. These issues are also encountered by those who care for people with cancer. Whether caring in a personal or professional capacity, carers also require support to maintain functioning in their roles as carers. This chapter specifically focuses upon those who care for people with cancer — the caregivers. This chapter will consider some of the issues caregivers are confronted with and identify supportive strategies that may be utilised to ensure that caregivers are supported and their needs are met. First, however, it is necessary to identify caregivers and to define key terms.

## DEFINING KEY TERMS

Caregiver is a conceptually broad term which can encompass parents, children, siblings, physicians, nurses, friends, physiotherapists, social workers, volunteers — the list is seemingly endless. In this chapter 'caregiver' will be used to mean only significant others and nurses. Significant others are those who share a significant personal relationship with the oncology client. Significant others may include individuals connected to the client by heredity and/or marriage. Significant others may also include nonmarital partners, fostered children, neighbours and friends. Significant others are therefore a group of people defined by the personal relationship they share with the client.

In this chapter 'nurses' means registered nurses who practise in oncology/haematology and provide professional nursing care for oncology

175

clients and significant others. Both institutionally based and community-based practitioners are included in this group

The 'client' is the person with cancer.

# VARIOUS ISSUES ENCOUNTERED BY ONCOLOGY NURSES AS CARERS

## Economic constraints and increased workloads

Nursing's role in today's health care is becoming increasingly difficult. Modern Western health care has adopted the Western industrial society ideologies that aim to generate monetary gain through productivity. As part of modern industrial society, Western hospitals are being held accountable for time and money spent on client care and are striving for efficiency and cost effectiveness (al Qadhi, 1996). Nursing potentially challenges these ideologies. Quality nursing care involves actions that produce no observable outcome and therefore are conceptually difficult to cost. What is the monetary value of sitting with a man as his wife dies of breast cancer? What is the cost of comforting parents as their son dies from acute myeloblastic leukaemia? In the drive for economic efficiency nurses' work is being scrutinised more and more. Nurses' workloads are increasing as each nurse is expected to take care of more clients. Observable, quantifiable nursing tasks, e.g. drug administration, can be costed in terms of time and resources consumed and are therefore taking priority over the qualitative concerns of caring and support. Although quantifiable tasks are elements of nursing care, less time is being devoted to qualitative concerns of caring (al Qadhi, 1996). In the drive for economic efficiency, opportunities for nurses to simply 'be' with clients are becoming rarer thus the caregiver role of nurses is being eroded.

Unfortunately, for oncology nurses, who value particularly the qualitative aspects of quality practice, the increasing lack of opportunities to comfort and support clients and significant others can result in increased job dissatisfaction.

## Grief

Nurses who work with clients suffering chronic and life-threatening illnesses are consistently surrounded by the possibility of client death. When a client dies nurses feel the impacts and grief in the loss of the therapeutic relationship that has developed over the course of the client's illness. However, much of nurses' response to the client's death is overlooked as the nurses aim to comfort and support significant others. Problems can arise when the demands of professional conduct discourage expressions of sadness.

When nurses experience grief and loss in a professional capacity, they too need to express feelings of sadness and/or relief without discouragement or judgment from their colleagues. The effects of loss and grief can be cumulative for nurses and, when not expressed, can affect nurses' ability to work and function efficiently, appropriately and professionally. Consequently the combination of work demands and cumulative grief can result in work dissatisfaction, lethargy, absenteeism, high staff turnover and burnout (al Qadhi, 1996). In such circumstances nurses' role of caregiver is diminished. As professionals, nurses require and deserve appropriate mechanisms through which to debrief and express their needs and emotions. Support mechanisms are suggested in the following sections.

# SUPPORT FOR NURSES AS CAREGIVERS

Several support mechanisms for oncology nurses have been identified in the clinical arena. However, the responsibility for support of oncology nurses is twofold, shared equally by the facility in which the nurses work and by oncology nurses themselves. Both nurses and the facility must recognise and be knowledgeable about the issues involved in caring for oncology clients before appropriate supportive strategies can be instigated. The following suggestions have been offered in support of oncology nurses.

## Maintain good health

The demands of shiftwork often result in irregular sleep, poor eating habits, lack of exercise and stress. These are factors that contribute to irritability, tiredness and poor health. Under these circumstances nurses' ability to be sensitive to the needs of their clients and therefore practise appropriately is diminished. It is important for nurses to eat well, exercise regularly and obtain sufficient sleep. Although these suggestions are common sense, they are important in maintaining physical, emotional and psychological health. By caring for their own health nurses equip themselves better to support and care for themselves and their clients in the workplace.

## Acknowledge the emotional impact of caring for oncology clients and their significant others

Caring for oncology clients and their significant others is complex and can often be difficult and demanding. It may appear that the oncology nurses' role is solely to care for terminally ill clients and their grieving significant others. It is important for nurses to understand that in caring for oncology clients and significant others they expose themselves to the risk of encountering grief on a personal and professional level. It is also important for nurses to understand that grief cannot be resolved unless it is recognised and acknowledged. If nurses assume that they are immune to the effects of grief at work, they are underestimating the potential impacts on their work and job satisfaction. In a specialty area such as oncology, nurses must be aware that they too are at risk of feeling the impact of loss and grief.

# Share responsibility

The responsibility of recognising the potential effects of grief in oncology nurses is twofold. Individual nurses must become familiar with their own attitudes to death and suffering and with their responses to them. Nurses must recognise their limits and be able to seek help and assistance when required. It is also the responsibility of nurses to recognise the effects of grief in their colleagues and to understand their need for support. Support must be offered readily and in the absence of criticism. Support may be offered in several ways: providing a shoulder to cry on, being someone to talk to or offering to take on part of the workload in order for a colleague to take an unplanned break, especially after the death of a client. Opportunities to offer support to colleagues are endless and range from simple gestures to more time-consuming, complex tasks. Collegial support is crucial to ensure that oncology wards foster an environment that supports nurses, thus enhancing their ability to care appropriately for oncology clients.

It is also the responsibility of nurse managers, associate nurse managers and clinical nurse specialists to recognise the potential for staff to experience grief and to acknowledge that the effects of grief are potentially cumulative. They must endeavour to create a working environment in which nursing staff feel supported and free to seek assistance and support without fear of criticism.

# Encourage managers to be accessible

Managers must be accessible to nursing staff. Accessibility demonstrates support through availability and indicates that managers are willing to discuss issues and take an active interest in their staff. Managers must also be able to communicate effectively with each staff member in order to assess their needs. This can be difficult and requires managers to tailor their communication style and technique to help them understand the needs of individual staff members.

# Continue with education

Inservice education is also demonstrative of support for nurses. Through education nurses are given the tools to be able to recognise issues as they arise. Through education nurses are also provided with skills and strategies to address these issues and resolve them appropriately for themselves and their colleagues.

# Debrief

Debriefing sessions conducted by counsellors are useful tools in providing an environment in which nursing staff feel supported in discussing and resolving issues associated with their work. These sessions may be conducted regularly or as the need arises. Managers are in a unique position to assess the needs of nursing staff through observation or discussion to facilitate debriefing sessions.

The opportunity to debrief can also be offered less formally. Some nurses will prefer to have a shoulder to cry on rather than a debriefing within a group session. Displaying concern and support in this manner will promote a working environment that is conducive to peer support.

## Maintain a professional relationship with clients

When nursing paradigms encourage consistency of care and promote relationship development between nurse and client (primary nursing) the impact of the client's illness and occasionally death has strong ramifications for the nurse. Relationships between nurses and clients can foster trust, communication, even friendship. Nurses need to be aware that the development of the relationship may leave them emotionally vulnerable in the event of the client's death, thus increasing their grief. It is important to maintain a relationship that is professional and client centred. Nurses must set clear, definable boundaries in which the nurse–client relationship may develop. When these boundaries are observed, the effects of loss and grief will not be avoided but their impact may be minimised (al Qadhi, 1996).

## Develop support networks

It is important for oncology nurses at all levels to develop support networks both at work and at home. The workplace may offer formal support groups and debriefing sessions. Colleagues are also valuable sources of support. They are familiar with issues involved in caring for oncology clients and their significant others and they are familiar with professional and personal difficulties encountered at ward level.

At home it is important to have people with whom to discuss difficulties, problems and issues. They may be partners, family members or friends who may not be associated with the world of nursing. They may offer different perspectives and coping mechanisms and are important sources of comfort, support and security. It is important that nurses foster these relationships as they offer valuable sources of support that may otherwise be unavailable.

## Seek help

Nurses who are inexperienced in oncology nursing are bombarded with treatment regimes which can be complicated and potentially dangerous to clients and staff. Similarly nurses confront many issues between a client and the client's significant others, issues that are physically and emotionally intense. Nurses can become easily overwhelmed. When nurses feel overwhelmed they experience isolation and frustration that jeopardises job satisfaction and professional practice (Puckett et al., 1996). It is imperative that nurses recognise their needs for support and seek them out. Often experienced peers and senior nursing staff are an excellent source of knowledge and can offer valuable support. However, they too are busy and may be unaware of the need for support of other nurses. Nurses must develop confidence in their ability to seek guidance. If work environments are conducive to peer support, the task is made easier. However if the work environment is intolerant of nurses who voice their needs, seeking support and guidance can often be difficult. Remember, as professionals, nurses are accountable for their actions. It is therefore imperative that help and guidance is sought when needed to maintain safe nursing practice and, often, sanity.

## Have fun

Although oncology/haematology nursing is challenging and often difficult, it can be immensely satisfying and enjoyable. While at work it is important to focus upon the professional and personal value of caring for people with cancer and their significant others. Nurses should take pride in the importance of the comfort and support they afford their clients. It is also important that nurses understand that tokens of gratitude offered by clients and significant others are well deserved and genuine gestures of appreciation in a job that can often appear thankless.

After work, nurses should treat themselves to simple pleasures. Things like eating fish and chips on the beach, having a drink with friends, going for walks, relaxing with a book or watching a favourite movie are rewards for a difficult job that has been done well. Relaxation and recognition of the need for small rewards are vital for nurses in stress relief and maintaining perspective of their work and its value to the community.

# VARIOUS ISSUES ENCOUNTERED BY SIGNIFICANT OTHERS AS CARERS

To many in the community a diagnosis of cancer is a death sentence. The change to the clients' perceptions of themselves, their health status and their mortality is shared by their significant others who are also profoundly affected. The issues encountered by significant others impact upon every facet of their lives when they are confronted with the possibility that the one they love requires extensive, often radical treatment the curative effects of which cannot be guaranteed. Like the client, significant others are confronted with issues that arise from the moment of diagnosis. These issues are varied and dependent on several factors, but they may revolve around grief, confronting mortality, fear, uncertainty, the change or loss of relationships, financial difficulties, isolation, guilt — the list seems unending. When caring for significant others it is imperative for oncology nurses to understand that the client and significant others are in a state of crisis and that there is no uniform progression of emotional change that significant others endure. The nature of the relationships between the client and significant others also impacts on the response of significant others; it is important for nurses to understand that each relationship is unique. There are also some particular ways that nurses can interact with and support significant others both when the client is ill and if the client has died.

# SUPPORT FOR SIGNIFICANT OTHERS AS CAREGIVERS

Although nurses' contact with significant others generally coincides with the admission of the client to hospital, significant others require support throughout the client's admission and after the client has been discharged or has died. The client's hospital admission offers nurses an excellent opportunity to assess significant others and identify issues with which support is required. Significant others may require support within the hospital setting and also in the community. It is therefore important that significant others' needs for support be identified immediately to ensure that support mechanisms are instituted promptly.

## Ensure accessibility to the client on admission to hospital

Include significant others in the admission of the client. This offers significant others an opportunity to be oriented to the ward, the hospital and the services offered. Provide significant others with telephone numbers of the facility, the ward and/or the client's bedside telephone. Hospital and ward policies will differ regarding the provision of telephone numbers so it is important to be familiar with such policies. Be sure to obtain the telephone numbers of the appropriate people and negotiate with them and the client circumstances and times of day and night in which they can be contacted. Also advise significant others and the client of visiting hours. These will also vary according to hospital and ward. It is important for significant others to have access to their loved ones. By obtaining and providing telephone numbers and advising significant others of visiting hours, nurses demonstrate that significant others have access to and are accessible by the client. In turn anxieties pertaining to separation from the client are acknowledged and addressed.

If the client is being cared for at home, ensure that significant others have the relevant contact numbers of community nurses to ensure that support is always available. Advise significant others of the hours of operation of community-based services and provide them with alternative contact numbers if out-of-hours assistance is necessary.

## Communicate effectively

Communication is one of the most important supportive strategies nurses can offer significant others. Everything nurses say and do communicates messages to both clients and significant others. It is important however to understand that communication is influenced by several factors. When speaking to significant others it is important to understand that they may be stressed, fearful and apprehensive which may influence their ability to comprehend and fully understand the information they are receiving about the client. Therefore, when speaking to significant others be concise and avoid technical and medical language. This will help to reduce confusion and misunderstanding. Also avoid the use of euphemistic language. There is a danger that euphemistic language may lead to confusion, especially if significant others are very young, distressed and/or from non-English-speaking backgrounds (Brown, 1995; Mian, 1990; Sinclair, 1996). For example, it is preferable to say that a client has died rather than 'passed on'.

Always be honest. If it is inappropriate for nurses to discuss medical components of the client's condition, significant others should be referred to the appropriate people. If nurses are unsure or unclear about aspects of treatment or the disease, they must always endeavour to refer significant others to colleagues who are able to offer accurate information. It is every nurse's responsibility to ensure that significant others have access to correct and accurate information. Nurses should not be afraid to acknowledge their limitations. It is preferable to do this rather than misinform significant others.

Sinclair (1996) identifies supportive nonverbal communication techniques such as facial expression, touch, eye contact and presencing. Touch, for example, can be a strong nonverbal communicator of concern and support as illustrated in the following example:

> . . . the only thing I could do for her was, well at that stage I just hugged her while he died and he died (Sinclair, 1996:32).

This example demonstrates that often when interacting with significant others there is little that can be said. It is sometimes preferable to demonstrate support nonverbally rather than offer platitudes which can be meaningless and detrimental to the care of significant others.

Similarly simply 'being there' communicates support and reassurance for significant others. Referred to as 'presencing', nurses' being present is indicative of their willingness to help and demonstrates their availability to care for the client and significant others (Benner, 1984). Presencing is an effective communicator of support in the latter stages of the client's illness when they may be uncomprehending or unconscious. At these times the client's impending death becomes a reality for significant others who are experiencing fear, uncertainty and grief. There is often little that can be said to comfort significant others at this time and nurses should avoid platitudes which are often glib and meaningless. Simply being there effectively communicates support.

Benner (1984), however, warns that, although nonverbal communication is an important communicator of support, it must be used with discretion. Touch, hugging, presencing, facial expressions and eye contact, for example, are sensitive to cultural, religious and personal interpretation. Ensuring that elements of nonverbal communication are not misinterpreted by significant others can be difficult. However, if they are employed sensitively in response to the needs of significant others, messages of support and reassurance will often be relayed.

## Assess the needs of significant others and refer them on

Assessing the needs of significant others is vital if nurses are to support them appropriately. Nursing assessments should be a continuous process as the needs of significant others change over time. Always ask them how they are coping at home. They may be experiencing difficulties with finances and the daily routines of managing a home. Social workers are a valuable resource who can arrange assistance with money, accommodation, travel, housework, meals etc. Be aware of hospital-based and community support groups who specialise in assisting significant others of oncology clients. Nurses are often able to arrange meetings between group facilitators and significant others who are experiencing difficulties. Psychologists and pastoral care workers are also valuable resources to be aware of for those who are encountering emotional, psychological and spiritual issues. The needs of significant others are multifaceted and often require assistance of allied health professionals. Be familiar with the allied support services and utilise them frequently.

## Provide education and information

Significant others are often unfamiliar with disease physiology, progression, symptoms, treatment options and side effects. They will require education which, as Benner (1984) states, is an important function of the nurses' supportive role. Significant others' ability to comprehend and process information may be affected by their emotional and psychological state. When educating significant others, keep explanations as concise as possible and avoid the use of technical language. Always encourage them to ask questions. Remember to refer them to colleagues when the accuracy of information or the appropriateness of subject matter is uncertain.

## Encourage interaction with clients at all times

Always encourage significant others to interact with the client. It is important that the relationship between the client and significant others be supported and encouraged to continue in circumstances that impose change upon individuals and their relationships. By encouraging significant others to interact with the client and take part in the care, nurses are demonstrating respect and support for the client, the significant others and the relationship they share. For clients at the end stages of the disease, interaction between them and significant others is particularly important. The relationship in these circumstances will soon be ended by the death of the client and every moment and action significant others share with the client is important. Offer significant others the opportunity to assist in providing nursing care and always provide them with opportunities to be alone with the client. As death becomes imminent, offer significant others the opportunity to stay overnight with the client. However, be sure that this is appropriate and consistent with hospital policy. As the client is dying, encourage significant others to hold the client's hand, touch their face, hug and kiss the client. At this stage the nurses' role should be primarily supportive. Do not be intrusive. Interact with the client and significant others in response to their needs.

When the client has died allow significant others to stay with the client for as long as they need if it is appropriate to do so. Offer them the opportunity to wash the client and even prepare the client for the mortuary. This is not as gruesome as it sounds. Remember this is the last opportunity significant others have to see, touch, be with and farewell the client before the funeral. These moments are important for significant others to acknowledge that death has occurred and to begin or continue grieving (Mian, 1993; Dyer, 1993). Significant others will cherish their final moments with the client and it is important that nurses provide the opportunity for them to be involved with the client for as long as they require.

## Encourage significant others to treat themselves

It is important that significant others have a break from the intensity of the client's illness. Encourage them to treat themselves to the pleasures of daily life that they once took for granted. If the client is hospitalised, suggest a cafe for lunch, encourage them to see a film, let them know of nearby parks and gardens. Where possible obtain a contact phone number and reassure significant others they will be contacted if necessary.

If the client is being cared for at home with the aid of support services, every encouragement must be offered to significant others to pursue simple pleasures. Where possible encourage significant others to care for the client on a roster system so that each person is able to pursue activities that offer relief and pleasure. It is important that significant others maintain a sense of normality and relief from the responsibility of caring for a loved one with cancer.

## CONCLUSION

Caring for a person with cancer is challenging, at times difficult, but often rewarding. Like clients, carers are confronted with issues pertaining to death, grief, mortality and change. Whether carers are professional (nurses) or personal (significant others) they too require support and encouragement in order to support the client to the best of their abilities. As nurses it is our responsibility to ensure that significant others are fully supported during the client's illness and, often, death. Significant others will often need support from many sources in order for them to function at their optimum level. As nurses we are in an excellent and powerful position to ensure their needs are accurately assessed and that they receive the support they need.

We, as nurses, also have a responsibility to each other to ensure that we receive the necessary support that allows us to facilitate the professional care of our clients and their significant others. This may take the form of education, debriefing sessions or simply a shoulder to cry on. Ultimately, however, it is the responsibility of each nurse individually to make our needs heard and to seek the support we require.

This chapter has offered practical suggestions that nurses may utilise to support themselves, each other and significant others. Some are oriented toward the self, others are suggested in support of others. If we offer and receive the support necessary to function, care of the oncology client, although challenging, will remain a rewarding and fulfilling experience.

# References

al Qadhi S (1996): *Managing Death and Bereavement: A Framework for Caring Organisations.* Great Britain: Bourne Press Ltd.

Benner P (1984): *From Novice to Expert. Excellence and Power in Clinical Nursing Practice.* Sydney: Addison-Wesley Publishing Company.

Brown B (1995): Saying goodbye. *American Journal of Nursing* 95 3: 61–64.

Dyer I (1993): Breaking the news: Informing visitors that a patient has died. *Intensive and Critical Care Nursing* 9: 2–10.

Faulkner A (1995): *Working with Bereaved People.* Melbourne: Churchill Livingstone.

Mian P (1990): Sudden bereavement: Nursing interventions in the ED. *Critical Care Nurse* 10 1: 30–41.

Puckett P, Hinds P, Milligan M (1996): Who supports you when your patient dies? *RN* 59 10: 48–50, 52–53.

Raphael B (1990): *The Anatomy of Bereavement. A Handbook for the Caring Professions.* Great Britain: Routledge.

Sinclair C (1996): How nurses interact with significant others when an oncology patient dies. BN (Honours) thesis, University of Melbourne.

Smith S, Pennells M (1995): *Interventions with Bereaved Children.* London: Jessica Kingsley Publishers Ltd.

Starck J, McGovern J (1992): *The Hidden Dimensions of Illness: Human Suffering.* New York: National League for Nursing Press.

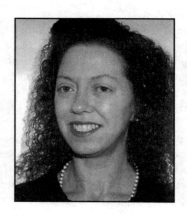

### LERA O'CONNOR
**Registered Nurse, Bachelor of Nursing Education**

Lera O'Connor completed her nursing training at the College of Nursing, Australia, in 1978. An interest in chronic disease led her to a primary focus on cancer so Lera has spent the last ten years working at the Peter MacCallum Cancer Institute in Melbourne. Most recently Lera has been working as a primary nurse in the community and has developed a specific interest in the area of cancer pain control.

Lera completed her nursing education degree in 1985 and since then has been involved in teaching. For three years she was the course coordinator of the cancer nursing course held at 'Peter Mac' before returning to full-time clinical nursing. She now teaches the pain control components of short-course programs and study days.

Lera is currently working as a project officer in the drug treatment services area with the Victorian state government and is completing a Master of Public Health at Monash University.

# Chapter 14

## *Multiculturalism — implications for cancer care*

This chapter presents a broad perspective on some of the problems that may be faced by people diagnosed with cancer who come from a cultural background that is different from that of the country in which they are living. Specific groups are not highlighted but general problems are discussed which may be relevant to many cultures. While the focus of the chapter is Australian society with particular examples drawn from the state of Victoria the implications are the same for any country which has welcomed many immigrants and particularly any country where the main language is some variety of English. The chapter is designed to raise your awareness of the complexities of nursing within a multicultural environment.

## OUR MULTICULTURAL SOCIETY

Australian society is comprised of people from more than 100 countries, speaking some 160 languages. Cultural groups include people from Europe, North and South America, Asia and Africa. In the state of Victoria at least 80 ethnic community organisations, and another 22 specifically for the elderly, serve this increasingly diverse population (Multicultural Affairs Unit, 1996).

It has been said that 'the great divide between humans and animals is culture' (Murray et al., 1985:3). What is meant by the word 'culture'? It can be defined as a group's 'design for living', a shared set of assumptions about the nature of the world. It is the sum total of the learned ways of doing, thinking, and feeling of a particular social group (Murray et al., 1985:4).

Within cultures there will be, on a smaller scale, subcultures. These groups can have values and beliefs quite different from those of the dominant culture, but still related in many ways. Subcultures may be defined around age, socioeconomic status, religion, education, occupation, or ethnic origin. Many subcultures abound in Australian society, and it is reasonable to expect a similar situation in all cultures. This means the practice of generalising about people on the basis of cultural background, or stereotyping, is likely to be inaccurate in many cases.

Cultural background impacts on all areas of life, and is expressed through both words and actions. A person's culture gives meaning and significance to their life. Aspects of culture include:

- values and value systems;

- beliefs; and

- ideologies (Kanitsaki, 1989).

Not all cultures have similar underlying characteristics. Some may appear less technological and more primitive in comparison to the technological Australian society. How may people from these cultures respond to biomedical interventions? How can a CT scan be explained adequately to a person whose belief systems are based in a traditional rural culture that does not use electricity? How do you describe the concept of ionising radiation to a person with no formal education who does not speak English? What expressions can give meaning to these concepts within another set of beliefs? These and other questions are examples of some of the complexities involved in caring for people with cancer from other cultures.

## HEALTH AND CULTURE

It is well accepted that health is a dynamic state influenced by many variables. Models of health have been proposed which help to explain the relationship between internal and external influences and health. These can be useful when trying to explain the influence of culture on a person's health.

One particular model describes health outcomes as a result of interactions between:

- genetic and biological characteristics;

- lifestyle, that is, personal behaviour such as smoking, alcohol consumption, diet, physical activity;

- the environment, including social and physical factors; and

- access to and use of health care services (Lalonde, 1974).

Whilst there has been some criticism of this model, it can serve as a useful basis on which to start exploring the implications of cultural variations for the health of individuals. The model recognises that the interplay of many variables will impact on a person's health status. It encompasses both environmental and individual factors, which are important when conceptualising cancer development.

The model can also be used as a framework on which to base health information, assessing the impact of culturally influenced lifestyle factors on the diagnosis and management of disease. A person and their family may be coping with the dual problems of a cancer diagnosis and settling into a new environment which is very likely to present different values from the environment they have known. There may be mixed feelings of grief, bewilderment, and inadequacy in adjusting to a new country (Hassan et al., 1985:278). There may also be new learning required; learning to handle the anxiety of family separations, establishing new social links, mastering a new language and adjusting to the health system into which they have been thrown. These tasks become increasingly difficult with advancing age or poor health.

People in minority cultures face problems, especially in the areas of access to and equitable use of health care services. This is particularly evident, in an English-speaking country, for those people from a non-English-speaking background (NESB).

In Victoria, factors that have been identified which contribute to inequities in the use of health care services include:

- lack of knowledge of services;

- lack of English language proficiency;

- inadequate targeting of NESB clients by individual agencies;

- cultural norms which preclude the use of certain services;

- geographic isolation;

- lack of awareness of staff in the health services to alternative cultural perspectives/practices; and

- standardised health care (as opposed to tailoring for those with differing needs) (Office of Multicultural Affairs, 1994).

Appropriate planning of the structure and delivery of health care services is one way to assist in overcoming many of these problems. In addition, the environment of individual health care agencies, a major responsibility of those working within them, must be empathetic to the varied needs of all their clients. This empathy will be reflected in the philosophy of each organisation and expressed through its mission statement.

# PERSPECTIVES ON ILLNESS: CULTURAL DIFFERENCES

Illness, pain (physical or emotional) and death are common life experiences confronting all people within all cultures at some stage. People develop 'rituals' to provide ways of dealing with life events such as illness and death. These serve important functions at an individual and societal level. Those rituals developed around death and grieving are a good example. How people respond to death depends upon the customs and traditions associated with their specific religion, belief and value systems, and the constructed relationship between life and death (Kanitsaki, 1989). Responses may vary greatly between traditional and more modern societies.

As humans, we attach particular meanings to these experiences that will ultimately be expressed in communication and behaviour. The meanings and implications attached to a particular illness will be screened through cultural beliefs.

Think about an Anglo-Saxon response to illness. It is based in a culture that values health, strength and productivity so illness is viewed as a condition to be prevented if possible. The person faced with an incurable illness often has difficulty accepting that the illness is incurable. Resignation is not a highly prized virtue in an activity-oriented society. Among other concerns, individuals express fears of 'being a burden', not unusual in an environment which stresses independence.

If one does become ill, it is usual to seek medical advice, and to comply with the advice given in order to get well. Getting back to work is seen as therapeutic in many cases. In relation to a cancer diagnosis, one is expected to accept the diagnosis, tolerate treatments (usually directed by a cancer specialist), and strive for the maintenance of independence throughout the process.

Age will influence attitudes to the development of cancer. How much easier it is to accept a cancer diagnosis in a 70-year old than a seven-year old. In our culture, age, illness and disability belong together.

What is the attitude of health professionals to those who cannot be cured? How do we, as nurses, deal with people in this environment? Do we encourage the search for a cure that does not exist to prolong hope? Or do we assist the person to accept the inevitable? How will acute episodes of illness be treated within the context of a terminal disease? Will medical treatment be sought for the person with acute asthma who has a prognosis of less than six months due to a malignancy?

The answers you provide to the questions posed are (in part) a reflection of your philosophy on illness, which often has its basis in cultural values. Attitudes will ultimately be expressed in behaviours, and, as nurses, we may find our care becomes a reflection of personal philosophy. This may or may not be congruent with the patient's perspective, and in many cases, may differ markedly from that person's understanding and needs in a particular situation.

The potential for miscommunication and misunderstanding on the part of both parties is high when the nurse and the patient come from two outwardly different cultures. The patient may be viewed as an immigrant entering a different culture, the biomedical culture (Underwood and Grey, 1987). This culture is based on Western models of science, and has the tendency to separate disease from the individual and their social context. This is not the basis for many other cultures' views of disease.

Cancer conjures up many meanings, negative in most cultures. A person's cultural beliefs may or may not be accurate or helpful, and may or may not lead to positive coping and adaptation to both the disease and planned treatments. Cultural practices, such as periods of fasting and the use of medicinal herbs, may be at odds with the goals of cancer management directed by an oncologist trained in Western medicine. Fasting may be detrimental to a person in whom nutritional status is already a problem, and some herbs may lead to colitis and diarrhoea. Situations such as these, where the benefits of various health care practices are culturally recognised, can lead to conflict between health care professionals and patients.

A focus on the different aspects of culture and their influences on health, illness, and health care practices was outlined initially by Madeleine Leininger in North America in the 1960s. She referred to transcultural or cross-cultural nursing, with a goal of providing culture-specific nursing care to people (Leininger, 1978). She outlined the concept of 'cultural relativity' (behaviour that is appropriate in one culture may not be appropriate in another) versus ethnocentrism (belief that one's own set of behaviours is best for everyone).

This view has clear implications for clinical practice and the nurse–patient relationship. Stereotyping can be seen as an act of disrespect, and can be the beginning of a process of desensitisation towards people of particular cultural groups. Think back to the discussion on subcultures at the beginning of this chapter and realise how complex and difficult it is to categorise any person, and what a mistake it is to do so. When one becomes used to treating people in a certain way this becomes the norm, but that can have negative consequences (Loff, 1994).

One can see the importance of nurses understanding each patient's meaning of a cancer diagnosis. How does that patient and their family perceive cancer? Is the diagnosis linked to feelings of anxiety, hopelessness, fear of death? What are the long-term implications of this?

What treatments or health care practices would a culture-specific practitioner usually prescribe? Can these be incorporated into the plan of care? What is the role of various family members in caring for a sick or dying person at home? Thinking about these questions and trying to find the best answers can greatly enhance the quality and appropriateness of care given to a person from a different cultural background.

# CROSS-CULTURAL COMMUNICATION

Communication is the basis of all human interactions. In any English-speaking country, the problems faced by people from a non-English-speaking background may be immense. In Victoria, Australia, only about 40 per cent of NESB women over 65 years report being able to speak English well or very well, and 53 per cent of NESB men report similar proficiency (Ethnic Affairs Unit, 1995a:8). Due to recency of arrival and different grammatical and pronunciation rules, the problem may be more severe for those speaking some Asian languages. For example, among elderly Victorians, only 7 per cent of those born in Vietnam report being able to speak English well or very well (Ethnic Affairs Unit, 1995a:8). Language differences may give a false impression about the intelligence of the person; English can be very difficult to master as a second language.

As nurses, observation and communication are the tools we use to ascertain the needs of those we are caring for. When messages are misinterpreted or misunderstood, communication breaks down. Causes of communication breakdown include:

- use of stereotypes and preconceptions;

- failure to explore the full meaning of words and behaviour;

- failure to understand that some people answer 'yes' to a question to please the questioner without truly understanding what is being asked;

- failure to listen;

- cliches and automatic responses; and

- failure to interrupt conversation for clarification (Travelbee, 1971).

It is not surprising that communication is often a major obstacle in dealing with the health care system and those working within that system. Communication techniques such as reflection, sharing perceptions, eye contact, and touch may not be appropriate for all cultures and the degree of physical proximity and touch which is comfortable will vary among cultures.

The onus for overcoming communication barriers is on the treating health professionals. Service delivery, including quality of the service, remains the responsibility of the service provider.

# WORKING WITH INTERPRETERS AND TRANSLATORS

Informed decision-making can only take place in an environment where all parties are participating equally. In English-speaking countries the inability to understand English to a proficient level can make this process impossible, and can lead to a lack of informed consent. Dependence rather than autonomy is fostered in this situation.

A professional interpreter (spoken communication) or translator (written communication) can make a great deal of difference to the quality of services the person from a non-English-speaking background receives, and can ensure true informed consent. Interpreters and translators will strive to ensure that information is received and conveyed accurately, and will often reduce the time required to achieve this aim.

Translated information is an effective way of improving communication and, in some cases, can reduce the need for interpreters. Translations of common questions and phrases pertaining to specific clinical situations can be photocopied and used for multiple patients. Commonly used forms can also be translated into relevant community languages. However, it is important to be aware that some people may be unable to read the language that they speak or the written language of their birthplace may not be the same as the dialect they speak, that is, they may be illiterate in their own language.

It is clear that the need for interpreters is paramount but there is a shortage of them, particularly for the special needs of women and the elderly. Reluctance to ask for interpreters (especially by women) has been shown to be a problem; many are unlikely to request an interpreter for fear of being considered impolite, and their request being rejected (Ethnic Affairs Unit, 1995a:10). This makes many people dependent on the 'goodwill' of the organisation with which they are dealing.

An interpreter is needed in all situations when the patient's English language skills are insufficient for the complexity of communication required. The interpreter does not become involved in any way with the information being handled, only seeking clarification of information as required. In Australia not all language groups have accredited interpreters, but communities often have recognised members who can function in this role. Face-to-face interpreters are preferred, but these must be booked in advance. This is not always practical, as some situations cannot be preplanned. Telephone interpreters are appropriate in these situations.

The use of family (especially children) or friends for interpreting is usually not appropriate. If clarification of appointments, medications, or other such information is sought, family members can be used, but otherwise an objective and noninvolved interpreter is required. Urgent situations, such as a sudden change in medical condition, are handled by the best means available at the time.

Agencies using interpreters should provide information on their correct use. The Ethnic Affairs Unit has produced a handy guide for working with interpreters which can be easily obtained (Ethnic Affairs Unit, 1995b).

It is not enough to think that the provision of interpreters is all that is required to offer culturally appropriate care. Refer back to our discussion on health and culture; many factors have to be taken into consideration. A climate of acceptance, open communication, and a desire to understand the problems faced by those not born in our society are all equally important.

## TRUTH TELLING AND INFORMED CONSENT

Major issues in cancer care relate to truth telling and informed consent (Kanitsaki, 1989). When analysed in light of different cultural considerations these can take on a whole new perspective. Different people and groups will respond to the word 'cancer' in various ways. Information must be given carefully, and in a culturally appropriate manner. For some cultural groups, telling the truth about a cancer diagnosis will be appropriate but for others it will not. This can present problems to health professionals from a predominantly Anglo-Saxon culture, where truth telling is considered of paramount importance.

Without making the mistake of stereotyping it is fair to say that the Greek culture provides an appropriate example here. Within this culture there is a collective family decision-making process, with family members considering they are in the best position to know what is in the patient's best interests (Kanitsaki, 1989). Upsetting this process can have harmful psychological consequences for the patient and their family. This is just one example of how the application of the cultural mores of the majority group within a society can be detrimental to other groups within that society.

It is neither possible nor practical to have a deep understanding of all cultures and subcultures and the individuals within them. The importance of individual assessment is highlighted here, with the nurse (and other members of the health care team) having a responsibility to ascertain what is appropriate for each patient and his or her family in specific situations.

# CROSS-CULTURAL SENSITIVITY

Australia is a typical example of all English-speaking countries in having as part of its society a number of minority groups with alternative cultures. Being aware of alternative cultures provides a starting point for communication in the relationship between an individual nurse and his/her patient from another culture.

A recognition and acceptance of another person's cultural beliefs and behaviours (including language) forms the basis for a meaningful nurse–patient relationship. Showing an understanding, no matter how limited, of the culture and dialects of any group will enhance acceptance and care of that person. Ethnocentric behaviour on the part of health care team members is likely to promote feelings of alienation and isolation in the person being cared for, and will not promote therapeutic relationships.

Autonomy and self-determination allow individuals and communities to improve the quality of their health (and life) through the process of empowerment. It is an action principle guiding activities and relationships necessary in health care, for example the ability to access appropriate resources necessary for health. Education and self-determination go hand in hand, as informed decision-making is an essential component of autonomy. Autonomy is one step closer when there is an understanding of the workings of the health care system and one's place in it.

In Australia one can look to the indigenous people for an example here. Autonomy is seen by indigenous people as fundamental to improvements in their health and wellbeing (Anderson, 1994:34). In regard to health programs, a truly culturally appropriate service for indigenous people will be community driven, with the values of that community incorporated into the design and implementation of the program (Anderson, 1994:34). The Aboriginal Health Services are examples of such programs. Most components of the Australian health care system do not cater so closely for multicultural communities.

Meaningful participation in decision-making regarding health care and treatments can promote self-determination in even a limited capacity. People can be assisted in navigating the health care system through the provision of appropriate assistance with and information about existing community resources.

# CONCLUSION

This chapter has raised many issues of which nurses must be aware when patients come from minority cultures. These issues are concerned not only with communication difficulties because of a poor understanding of the country's major language (English in Australia) but also the problems of dealing with cultural differences that cause tension between existing health care services and the expectations of people from minority cultures. An important part of the successful treatment of patients from minority cultures is to find ways in which the nurse and the patient can communicate effectively and can reach some degree of harmony so that the patient gains the maximum benefit from the health care system.

## References

Anderson I (1994): Health and human rights: The burden of racism. *Seminar proceedings: The continuum of health and human rights.* Melbourne: Macfarlane Burnet Centre for Medical Research.

Ethnic Affairs Unit (1995a): Speaking of Diversity . . . *Delivering Translating and Interpreting Services to Non-English Speaking Background Victorians.* Melbourne: Ethnic Affairs Unit, Department of the Premier and Cabinet.

Ethnic Affairs Unit (1995b): *Working with Interpreters: A Guide for Victorian Government Departments and Funded Agencies.* Melbourne: Ethnic Affairs Unit, Department of Premier and Cabinet.

Hassan R, Healy J, McKenna R, Hearst S (1985): Vietnamese Families. In Storer D (ed.): *Ethnic Family Values in Australia.* Australia: Prentice-Hall of Australia Pty Ltd, pp. 263–289.

Kanitsaki O (1989): Cross Cultural Sensitivity in Palliative Care. In: Hodder P, Turley A (eds): *The Creative Option of Palliative Care: A Manual for Health Professionals.* Melbourne: Melbourne Citymission, pp. 68–71.

Lalonde M (1974): *A New Perspective on the Health of Canadians.* Ottawa: Information Canada.

Leininger M (1978): *Transcultural Nursing: Concepts, Theories, and Practices.* New York: John Wiley.

Loff B (1994): Setting the scene: The health and human rights continuum. *Seminar proceedings: The continuum of health and human rights.* Melbourne: Macfarlane Burnet Centre for Medical Research.

Multicultural Affairs Unit (1996): Victorian *Multicultural Resources Directory.* Melbourne: Multicultural Affairs Unit.

Murray R, Zentner J, Samiezadi-Yazad C (1985): Spiritual and Religious Influences on the Person. In: *Nursing Assessment & Health Promotion Strategies Through the Life Span* (4th edn). Norwalk: Appleton & Lange.

Office of Multicultural Affairs (1994): *Achieving Access and Equity*. Canberra: Australian Government Publishing Service.

Travelbee J (1971): *Interpersonal Aspects of Nursing* (2nd edn). Philadelphia: FA Davis Company.

Underwood P, Gray D (1987): The Fragility of Our Sun: A Doctor Rediscovers the Cultural Wheel. In: Joske R, Segal W (eds): *Ways of Healing*. Australia: Penguin, pp. 29–46.

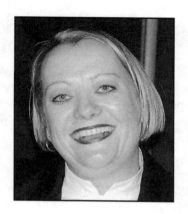

## MAREE CUDDIHY
**Registered Nurse; Registered Midwife; Bachelor of Nursing; Graduate Certificate Oncology Nursing, Marsden; Graduate Diploma of Advanced Nursing (Administration), La Trobe University; Master of Business, Royal Melbourne Institute of Technology; Member of the Royal College of Nursing, Australia; Fellow of the Williamson Community Leadership Program**
**Quality Coordinator, Peter MacCallum Cancer Institute, Melbourne**

Maree has spent most of her life working with people with cancer. She has experience in most areas of nursing including rural health care, clinical practice, nursing education, nursing administration and now quality improvement. She is enthusiastic about the future of nursing.

# Chapter 15

## *Exploring the boundaries of oncological nursing practice*

> *Time present and time past*
> *Are both perhaps present in time future,*
> *And time future contained in time past.*
> —T.S. Eliot in 'Burnt Norton' from Four Quartets

## HEALTH CARE IN AUSTRALIA IN THE 1990s

Health care, especially in public hospitals, seems to be a running sore for most governments. For too long their capacity to deal effectively with the problems in health has been restricted by the escalating cost of the system. The continuing growth in the cost of medical and pharmaceutical services, an increasingly aging population and a reduction in the numbers of people taking out private health insurance have restricted governments' capacity to deal with a broad range of problems. At the same time, the community's expectations of the health system have never been higher — the number of general practitioner visits per head has nearly doubled in the last 10 years, and Australia has one of the highest numbers of hospital admissions in the world (Health and Community Services, 1995).

Problems of health care reform are universal. In Australia, and probably in other developed countries, elements of the reform agenda appear to be based on:

* making better use of available resources;

* continuing microeconomic reform;

* encouraging real competition and service innovation in the health market; and

* clarifying management of the system between jurisdictions.

## Making better use of available resources

Increasingly governments are focusing efforts on health promotion and illness prevention. In Australia we have such examples as the National Cancer Control

Initiatives 1997–1998, VicHealth (in Victoria) which funds many health-promoting initiatives, and activities conducted through the Anti-Cancer Councils in all Australian states. Governments are also encouraging new funding and organisational arrangements for community and home-based care through such initiatives as post-acute care programs and coordinated care trials funded by the Commonwealth government.

## Continuing microeconomic reform

In Victoria the expansion of the inpatient 'activity-based funding', known as Casemix/DRG (diagnosis-related groupings) funding, to the non-inpatient setting through Victorian Ambulatory Care separations is continuing microeconomic reform within the health system. Several Australian state governments are moving to purchasing services only from accredited hospitals. It is not unrealistic to imagine that in the future activity-based funding will also apply to community-based organisations.

Bureaucracies are requesting from hospitals more activity-based, and quality-based, information which is then being made available to the public. This provides patients with information about variations between hospitals in order for patients to make informed choices about seeking health services, and provides governments with more comprehensive information on resource usage.

## Encouraging real competition and service innovation in the health market

Increasing options are available to governments to purchase services from both private and public hospitals, thus increasing competition between the sectors. Monopolies that existed previously in the public sector are being challenged by the emergence of new service products such as integrated health centres and more day procedure facilities.

## Clarifying management of the system between jurisdictions

To date reform in health care in Australia has been targeted largely at short-term budget solutions. Real reform will require broadly based performance agreements between the Commonwealth government and the states in order to stop duplication of services and cost shifting. For example, at the moment the state governments are responsible for inpatient funding and the Commonwealth government is mostly responsible for non-inpatient funding. Improving coordination at a service level remains complex because of a lack of incentives.

# THE SITUATION OVERSEAS

Evidence of the international trend in these areas can be seen from the following eloquent excerpt:

**Table 15.1 Characteristics of the emerging health care system in the USA**

The characteristics of the emerging health care system are:

**Orientation toward health**: Greater emphasis on prevention and wellness and greater expectation of individual responsibility for healthy behaviours.

**Population perspective:** New attention to risk factors affecting substantial segments of the community, including inaccessibility and physical and social environments.

**Intensive use of nformation**: Reliance on information systems to provide complete, easily assimilated patient information, as well as ready access to relevant information on current practice.

**Focus on the consumer:** Expectation and encouragement of patient partnerships in decisions related to treatment, facilitated by the availability of complete information on outcomes and partly evaluated by patient satisfaction.

**Knowledge of treatment outcomes:** Emphasis on the determination of the most effective treatment under different conditions and the dissemination of this information to those involved in treatment decisions.

**Constrained resources:** A pervasive concern for increasing costs, coupled with expanded use of mechanisms to control or limit available expenditures.

**Coordination of services:** Increased integration of providers, with a concomitant emphasis on teams to improve efficiency and effectiveness across all settings.

**Reconsideration of human values:** Careful assessment of the balance between the expanding capability of technology and the need for humane treatment.

**Expectations of accountability:** Growing scrutiny by a larger variety of payers, consumers, and regulators, coupled with more formally defined performance expectations.

**Growing interdependence:** Further integration of domestic issues of health, education, and public safety, combined with a growing awareness of the importance of US health care in a global context.

(Adapted from O'Neil E, 1993, Health professions education for the future: Schools in service to the Nation, San Fransico, CA: Pew Health Professions Commission. Reprinted for this book from Hamric A, Spross J and Hanson C, 1996, *Advanced Nursing Practice*, published by W.B. Saunders Company, p. 64)

Each of the above characteristics provides opportunities for nurses and nursing, especially in the field of oncological nursing.

## A ROLE FOR NURSES?

The solutions to the problems outlined above do not lie just with nurses. However, since nurses still remain the largest single discipline in most health institutions, imagine the potential if nurses came together to lead the way in creating the future.

Nurses have been engaged in changing, adapting and expanding clinical practice roles for many years. The challenges and changes that nurses face today are a mere preparation for the future. As Hamric and associates (1996:252) assert:

> change not stability characterises the work in nursing and in health care, a formerly predictable field. Nurses at all levels and all settings must develop a working comfort with change in order to respond flexibly and plan effectively in ever-changing environments.

Those oncology nurses who have been in the field for a while should take a moment to reflect on the rapidity, constancy and increasing complexity of the new learning that is required for clinical reasoning. Where a facility is involved in clinical trials, the complexity and increased accountability seems doubled.

Porter (1995) points out, when discussing ambulatory oncology nursing practice, that the role of the oncology nurse varies widely in different organisations and settings, and even among settings in the one organisation. The role has been shaped primarily in response to the philosophy of the administrators and the medical staff and the education level of the nurses, as well as the nurses' experience or exposure to other settings. Porter (1995) says nurse activities are also affected by organisational budget resources and nursing leadership. For example, if reduction in the quality of care is palatable because management of the declining budget is the most important objective of the senior decision-makers, then the importance of the role of the registered nurse will diminish relative to less costly nurses, for example, Division 2 registered nurses (enrolled nurses) and personal care attendants. Therefore, given the continuing financial constraint, more so then ever before, it is essential that if nurses want to create their own future they must identify their contribution to patient care and articulate their interdependent role, not only in terms of health outcomes but also in terms of financial outcomes.

The biggest success factor towards or barrier against nurses establishing greater professional interdependence with their medical colleagues and acceptance by administrators is attitude. It is essential that nurses develop both an individual and a collective attitude of acceptance that today's health care system requires collaborative professional relationships and flexibility to change. In addition nurses need to be willing to hold up to scrutiny traditional practice patterns. The most important single challenge for nurses will be to cease defending functions and roles that are obsolete.

Stichler (1995:53) rightly contends that collaboration among the different health disciplines has never been more critical:

> Multiple disciplines converge on the patient and family to rapidly identify needs, implement and coordinate interventions, and plan for post discharge care in different settings.

This is all accomplished in the least amount of time and is driven by financial imperatives. Hence the management and coordination of the care process across settings — inpatient, non-inpatient, home-based care and different hospitals — is very important to prevent duplication of services like pathology and x-ray, but more importantly to ensure that the patient does not fall through gaps in the system and therefore not receive maximum health care. In addition, patient complexity alone necessitates that attention be given to collaboration with doctors. Doctors are ordering more complex treatments for patients who are more often moving between inpatient and non-inpatient settings. The complexity is not only physical but psychosocial, requiring considerable coordination. It is increasingly difficult for doctors to keep track of what has occurred with patients.

Stichler (1995:54) borrows from the field of psychology to define collaboration as:

> a specialised term for an interpersonal relationship that combines cooperation and sensitivity to the needs of another.

Collaboration between health care professionals must recognise the interdependence between disciplines and specialities and must value the input of others. By necessity this collaboration must be viewed as a developmental process that evolves as trust between team members grows and, ultimately, interdependent working relationships are realised. Writers generally (Hamric et al., 1996; Stichler, 1995; Moore, 1996) support the view that professional, and thus advanced clinical, competence by the nurse is fundamental in order for real physician–nurse collaboration to develop. Nurses at all levels in an organisation do, and should be encouraged to, develop opportunities to engage in professional interaction with doctors that lead to strong collaborative relationships. Collaboration often occurs through the model of:

- primary nursing at the bedside;

- participating in ward rounds;

- engaging in planning the patient's care; and

- reinforcing, in the formal manner, the doctor's understanding of the nurse's role in accomplishing the desired patient outcomes.

## ADVANCED PRACTICE NURSES

Advanced practice roles (nurse–doctor partnerships) are being developed in a variety of primary and acute settings not only in response to restrictions on medical staff work hours, the cost of employing more doctors and the difficulty in recruiting doctors to rural areas, but, more importantly, in response to the increased ability and education of nurses. Whilst the use of nurse practitioners or advanced practice nurses (APNs) is widespread, especially in North America, it is evolutionary in Australia. Nevertheless a number of APNs have developed unique and convincing roles, opening new opportunities for their colleagues (Smith, 1996). However, whilst many nurses are indeed pioneering a new career path for nurses in Australia, the information gleaned is rarely being shared with the profession (through conference and journal publication) nor is the value of such practices being measured. In general, many of these advances in practice are invisible, not only within the profession of nursing, but also within the health care system. Unless the nursing profession resolves this issue, the educational and professional development of nurses working in advanced roles will continue to flounder. This is an area in which it is critical that nurses communicate their experiences and ideas to their colleagues to enable role growth to occur and new models of practice to be found valuable.

The development of new roles in nursing will not be and indeed has not been without its pain. Amusingly, Stichler (1995) offers the Webster Dictionary definition of collaboration as a term '. . . used to describe a willing cooperation with one's enemy'. While this definition overstates the case (and is indeed a generalisation) it highlights the tension that can still exist between doctors and nurses.

# THE COMPETENT, ASSERTIVE NURSE

### Table 15.2 Tenets of an assertive philosophy

1. By standing up for our rights, we show we respect ourselves and achieve respect from other people.
2. By trying to govern our lives so as to never hurt anyone, we end up hurting ourselves and other people.
3. Sacrificing our rights usually results in destroying relationships or preventing ones from forming.
4. Not letting others know how we feel and what we think is a form or selfishness.
5. Sacrificing our rights usually results in training other people to mistreat us.
6. If we don't tell other people how their behaviours negatively affect us, we are denying them an opportunity to change their behaviour.
7. We can decide what is important to us; we do not have to suffer from the 'tyranny of the should and should not'.
8. When we do what we think is right for us, we feel better about ourselves and have more authentic and satisfying relationships with others.
9. We all have a natural right to courtesy and respect.
10. We all have a right to express ourselves as long as we don't violate the rights of others.
11. There is more to be gained from life by being free and able to stand up for ourselves and from honouring the same rights of other people.
12. When we are assertive, everyone involved usually benefits.

( From Jakubowski-Spector P, 1976, Self-assertive training procedures for women. In: D. Carter & E. Rawlings (eds), *Psychotherapy with women, Treatments towards equality*. Courtesy of Charles C. Thomas, Publisher, Springfield, Illinois. Reprinted for this book from Hamric A, Spross J and Hanson C, 1996, *Advanced Nursing Practice*, published by W.B. Saunders Company, p. 260.)

Hamric et al. (1996) suggest that among other competencies that nurses developing new roles need to demonstrate are appropriate assertive behaviours. Hamric et al. offer Jakubowski-Spector's (1976) 'tenets of assertive philosophy' as guiding principles. Obviously this philosophy needs to be upheld by a culture of open inquiry, curiosity, and high professional standards to list but a few essential characteristics.

# OPPORTUNITIES

At the beginning of this chapter I listed at least some elements of the reform agenda that are occurring in Australia today. The possibilities and opportunities for oncology nurses in the future lie, I believe, within the present reform and in what we know we have achieved in the past.

Successful outcomes of pilot projects like the Post-Acute Care Program, Hospital-in-the-Home and the Coordinated Care Trials that are taking place in Australia, amongst other Medicare reforms aimed at general practitioners and the funding of pharmaceuticals will **continue microeconomic reform**, heralding faster progression towards substitution from institutional to home-based care. It is also probable that, in Australia, governments will **clarify the management of the system between their jurisdictions.** Either the Commonwealth government will transfer responsibility to the states completely or, alternatively, the Commonwealth will retain responsibility with the states acting as service delivery agents. This will eliminate the different funding sources and the confusion that exists (often resulting in the patient losing out). Further, the next decade will witness additional erosion of the boundaries of hospital care by greater technological innovation (e.g. Telemedicine and the universal electronic record) which will enhance home-based care, same-day treatments and other alternatives to hospital inpatient care. Moreover, the **encouragement of real competition and service innovation in the health market** through the provision of more information to patients and the push towards privatisation will result in a more discriminating and probably more demanding patient (in terms of demanding value for money). If we stay with the proposition that has been posed, what remains (for nursing at least) is to **make better use of resources which are already available to the system.** Nurses are a resource available to the system. Nurses who have shown constantly throughout history how they have adapted and changed with the times can make a very significant contribution to the changes that are now being visited upon us.

The opportunities as I see them will still be influenced, as Porter (1995) pointed out, by the overarching philosophy of the institution and how that is enacted in staff relationships. If trust and mutual respect between professionals are not highly valued then expanding the boundaries of practice will not happen. However, on the other hand, where true collaboration does exist, even if it is only in pockets within the organisation, opportunities abound. Freedman in Stichler (1995) suggests that, in order to effect change, three components are required:

1.  There must be pressure for change (this is happening in Australia at both state and Commonwealth levels and, to varying degrees, in hospitals).

2.  Leaders must articulate clearly the direction for change (it is here that the institutions will vary, depending on culture and history).

3.  Those who are experiencing the change must have the desired skills or competencies.

The last point is an important one to be stressed. Nurses working within advanced practice roles experience a certain amount of autonomy. Patients are dependent upon them, so it follows that nurses have a professional responsibility to the community to be skilled, competent, knowledgeable and ethical about the practice they undertake. Therefore they must have a comprehensive knowledge base. Lin et al. (1993) advocate a formal learning program based on a cohesive relationship between the learner, the academic institutions and the work environment. Nurses need to be able to make direct application of the new knowledge in order to retain it. This is particularly so in the practice professions.

Areas for potential increased collaboration with doctors, and therefore opportunities, could include the following:

1.  Existing roles such as Chemotherapy Clinical Nurse Consultant and Transplant Nurse Coordinator could be extended to include:

    - full physical examinations;

    - ordering and interpreting laboratory and diagnostic imaging tests; and

    - working from standing orders and protocols to have a type of prescriptive authority.

These roles could also be extended to nurses undertaking advanced practice functions in ambulatory care and radiotherapy. Nurses working collaboratively with doctors would be responsible for specific cohorts of patients and, working within guidelines, for consulting with their medical peers when the patients' needs were beyond the nurses' level of competence. These roles would blend primary and acute care concerns resulting in constant caregivers across the continuum of patient care.

2.  It is possible for nurses to capitalise on the lack of early cancer detection screening in many centres. A US study described by Warren and Pohl (1990) revealed that, whilst physicians were aware of guidelines for early cancer detection, implementation was sporadic. It is possible that this is also the case in Australia. Clinics could be either nurse-run or collaborative practices that would include:

    - initial history and physical examination;

    - family history of cancer;

    - counselling on risk reduction;

- teaching cancer early warning signs;

- obtaining a smoking history;

- performing and teaching breast examination;

- referral for mammography;

- pap smears and vaginal examinations;

- testicular examination and teaching; and

- skin examination.

# CONCLUSION

This is an exciting time for nursing history, especially for advanced practice nurses. The changes and challenges facing nursing represent the future at our doorstep. The time to act is now. When opportunities present themselves, grasp them enthusiastically. When opportunities do not appear, work on the underpinning principles of trust and mutual respect based in sound clinical competence and see what happens.

***By our deeds they shall know us!!!***

## References

Eliot TS (1936): Burnt Norton, part 1, *Four Quartets*. In: Partington A (1993): *The Concise Oxford Dictionary of Quotations* (3rd edn). Oxford: Oxford University Press, p. 132.

Health and Community Services, Victoria, *Annual Report 1994-1995*.

Hamric A, Spross J, Hanson C (1996): *Advanced Nursing Practice: An Integrative Approach*. Philadelphia: W.B. Saunders.

Lin E, Aikin J, Bailey W, Fitzgerald B, Mings D, Mitchell S, Rigby B (1993): Improving ambulatory nursing practice. An innovative educational approach. *Cancer Nursing* 16 1: 53–62.

Porter H (1995): The effect of ambulatory oncology nursing practice models on health resource utilization: Part 1, Collaboration or compliance. *JONA* 25 1: 21–29.

Smith S (1996): Independent nurse practitioner advanced nursing practice in Brisbane, Australia. *Nursing Clinics of North America* pp. 519–563.

Stichler J (1995): Professional interdependence: The art of collaboration. *Advanced Practice Nursing Quarterly* 1 1: 153–161.

Warren B, Pohl J (1990): Cancer screening practices of nurse practitioners. *Cancer Nursing* 13 3: 143–151.

# SECTION FOUR

## *Examples of Australian research*

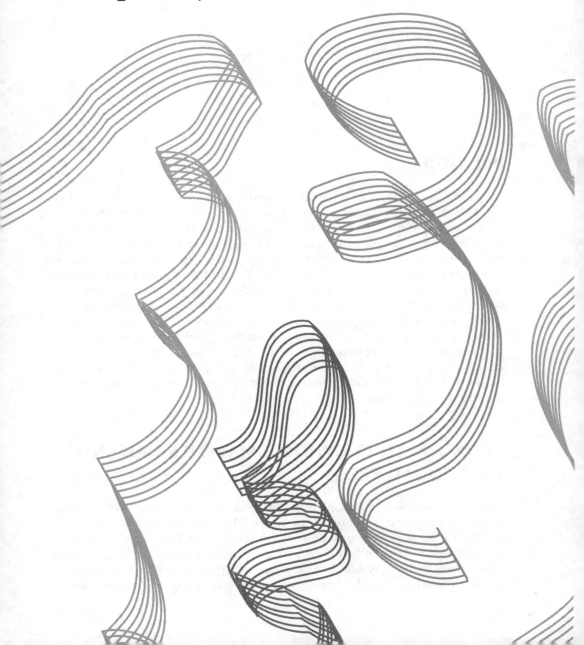

# Research piece A

## *Lymphoedema*
*Jennifer Green*

### PREAMBLE

Following the removal of a melanoma and a groin dissection at 29 years of age I developed lymphoedema in one of my legs. During childbirth, sporting activities, and some daily events my lymphoedema has caused me various problems which are difficult to deal with. As a nurse and therefore having a more 'privileged' access to the health care system I have been able to access management more easily than others. Yet my problems with lymphoedema remain significant. My own experience made me want to find out how others experience lymphoedema. This became the focus of my PhD thesis, which is where the data for this paper originates. The data which I have collected has made me very aware that people experience many more problems with lymphoedema than I had ever envisaged. It is a significant health care problem and, as the majority of lymphoedema is iatrogenically induced, it is a health care problem that demands to be addressed more by the health care system.

### LIVING WITH LYMPHOEDEMA: PHYSICAL AND EMOTIONAL NEEDS

Lymphoedema most commonly presents as a swelling of one or more limbs and/or the adjacent quadrant of the trunk. The pathosphysiology of lymphoedema is now clearly understood (Consensus Document of the International Society of Lymphology Executive Committee, 1995) and occurs when the lymphatic system is unable to drain protein and fluid from the tissues. Disturbance to the lymphatic system commonly occurs following surgical removal of, or radiotherapy to, lymph glands. These interventions are performed in an attempt to stop the spread of cancer from the breast, reproductive system or skin. Lymphoedema is often viewed (by those who do not have the condition) as a small price to pay for being 'cured' of cancer. With research indicating an increased rate of skin and breast cancer in our society it is anticipated that the incidence of lymphoedema may also increase.

For those affected by lymphoedema, the limb may become heavy, stiff and painful, and mobility may be reduced. The swollen limb causes disfigurement and is distressing to the person from physical, psychological and aesthetic points of view. It is a chronic and constant problem which the affected person must learn to manage and live with. The resultant stagnant high protein concentration in the tissues perpetuates an increased risk of infection. The infective episodes may further damage the lymphatics and lead to worsening oedema. The lymphoedema usually becomes more pronounced with advancing age. As lymphoedema is a persistent and generally irreversible condition it requires lifelong care and attention.

Several articles have been published over the past few years which address management of the lymphoedematous limb (Foldi, 1985; Foldi et al., 1985; Gray, 1987; Badger, 1987; Collard, 1990; Casley-Smith, 1992; Humble, 1995; Granda, 1994; Williams, 1997). These articles tend to assume that as long as the limb size is reduced and maintained lymphoedema is not a problem. No studies have been published which specifically address the problems individuals experience when living with lymphoedema.

# THE STUDY

The purpose of my study was to identify what people experience in their day-to-day lives as a result of living with lymphoedema and to ascertain their associated health care needs.

# METHOD

## Respondents

The respondents in this study were 157 people (135 females and 22 males) who subjectively claimed to have lymphoedema. Ages varied from less than 16 to greater than 75, with most being between 35 and 64. Over 80 per cent of the respondents had developed lymphoedema secondary to a medical or surgical intervention for the management of cancer. Of these, 59 per cent had been treated for breast cancer, 21 per cent for melanoma and 11.5 per cent for cancer of the uterus/cervix. The remaining 8.5 per cent had undergone lymph node biopsy.

## Instrument

A comprehensive questionnaire was developed to uncover

a)   demographic data and background information about lymphoedema;

b)   how much and how often reactions associated with lymphoedema were experienced; and

c)   the perceived needs of people with lymphoedema.

All questions relating to perceived needs included open-ended responses. Content validity was established through consulting with a panel of experts who regularly deal with people who have lymphoedema. A field test was conducted to further assess content validity as well as to assess face validity. The questionnaire was revised according to experiences in the pilot study.

## Procedure

It was the purpose of the study to survey respondents from Sydney and country areas of New South Wales. Respondents were accessed through an article placed in a the *Sun Herald* describing the study and calling for respondents. The questionnaire was mailed to 167 consenting respondents and yielded a 92 per cent response rate.

## Data analysis

The information obtained from the questionnaires was coded (to 92), stored on disk and analysed by a digital computer using the SPSS programs. Trends were identified from the qualitative data obtained.

## RESULTS

To determine how people are affected by lymphoedema the measurement of the physical/emotional reactions that people may experience as a result of having lymphoedema were identified and measured on a Likert scale. This scale used five points of 'agreement–disagreement' and a 'neither' category for those who were undecided about the symptoms of lymphoedema. A five-point-scale of 'never–always' and a 'sometimes' category was also used to determine how often people experienced the symptoms of lymphoedema. The frequency of responses to this scale are reported in Table A.1. The response of 'neither' or 'sometimes' (the middle point on the scale) is not indicated in this table and accounts for the gap between the total of responses and 100 per cent.

**Table A.1 Perceived sequelae of lymphoedema**

| | How Much It Fits Me | | How Often This Reaction Affects Me | |
|---|---|---|---|---|
| As a result of my swollen limb/s I experience: | Agree – Strongly Agree | Disagree – Strongly Disagree | Frequently – Always | Seldom – Never |
| · heaviness in the affected limb | 89% | 3% | | |
| · abnormal or funny sensation in the affected limb | 73% | 16% | 58% | 16% |
| · pain in the affected limb | 66% | 25% | 40% | 28% |
| · embarrassment | 66% | 20% | 37% | 36% |
| · joint stiffness in the affected limb | 64% | 24% | 39% | 35% |
| · decreased physical activity | 62% | 26% | 34% | 39% |
| · interference with daily living activities | 58% | 25% | 39% | 40% |
| · depression | 58% | 26% | 38% | 41% |
| · anxiety | 55% | 33% | 19% | 44% |
| · infection/inflammation in the affected limb | 51% | 29% | 28% | 47% |
| · decreased social activity | 42% | 35% | 17% | 58% |
| · a decrease in the frequency and quality of sexual relationships | 32% | 37% | 19% | 56% |

# Physical reactions

The most notable physical problem revealed was that the majority of respondents experienced heaviness in their affected limb a significant amount of the time. The disparity in experiences with limb heaviness, where 3 per cent strongly disagreed that they 'experience heaviness in their swollen limb' may be to do with the degree of swelling they had in their affected limb. Very mild and even unmeasurable degrees of lymphoedema were included, as the study accepted respondents on their subjective view that they had lymphoedema as this was considered to be more important than arbitrary difference in limb size (objective lymphoedema).

Activity limitation was experienced by over two-thirds of the respondents and resulted from one, or a combination of:

- increased weight of the limb,

- joint stiffness,

- pain and 'strange' sensations in the limb.

For those with lymphoedema of the arm, activity limitation included interferences with basic everyday activities such as dressing, washing, doing hair, cleaning, vacuuming, peeling potatoes, opening jars, buttering bread, bed making, hanging out clothes and carrying even light loads. For those with lymphoedema of the leg, sitting, walking or standing for a length of time caused pain, numbness, tingling, or a 'bursting' sensation in the leg. For many the necessary daily placement of the limb into the pressure garment was a struggle, especially in hot weather when the limb was larger.

Due to the physically debilitating effects of their lymphoedema one-quarter (n=40) of the respondents needed to give up work and a further 24 per cent (n=39) could cope with work only on a part-time basis.

Pain was, for some, the most debilitating symptom of lymphoedema. For many the intensity of the pain increased with exercise. One woman experienced such severe pain even at rest that she commented *'I just can't stand the pain much longer. I've given myself two more years, then I'm going to God. It's not the quantity of life, it's the quality of life . . .'*. Another respondent, a male in his early thirties with a young family, experienced such severe pain in his leg following surgery for melanoma that he had to take medical retirement from his teaching position.

Just over two-thirds of respondents (n=107) indicated that they did not socialise as much as they used to before the lymphoedema developed. Many indicated that they were unable to do the work associated with entertaining and therefore the ability to entertain was decreased. Respondents with lymphoedema of the leg identified the 'bursting' sensation experienced when sitting for a length of time in a movie theatre or at a restaurant as a reason for not socialising as much. For some the lymphoedema directly affected their ability to be involved in certain forms of socialising such as playing sport, bush walking or dancing.

People with leg oedema had the problem of not being able to buy shoes that fit. Others had problems finding clothes that would stretch over a swollen arm. The concern over physical appearance and the inability to wear appropriate clothing to certain functions created problems when wanting to socialise at more formal occasions — *'runners are the only shoes wide enough to fit'*.

## Emotional reactions

The disfigurement of breast surgery is not visible except in private situations. The disfigurement of lymphoedema in the leg or arm, and especially the hand can be quite visible. The visibility of lymphoedema and the resulting exposure of the person's encounter with cancer to unknown people caused many emotional reactions. Two-thirds of respondents (n=104) indicated that their swollen limb caused them to feel embarrassed and elicited comments such as *'Socially people stare; in change rooms and in public people ask me what is wrong with my hand'*. Over half of these coped with their embarrassment by hiding their affected limb behind clothing or staying at home. The perceived need to hide the limb behind clothing caused problems in summer when the wearing of long pants or long-sleeved shirts added to the discomfort of the heat. Others commented that they would not wear their compression garment out in public because, *'like a neon light'*, it drew attention to their lymphoedema.

Over half of the respondents (n=80) claimed that the lymphoedema caused them to become anxious. Not knowing just how bad the lymphoedema would become in the future was one of the causes of anxiety, eliciting comments such as, *'I worry about the lymphoedema becoming worse and controlling my life'*. Another cause of anxiety was the fear of the recurrence of cancer. The swollen limb reminded them constantly of their cancer experience. Not being able to perform simple tasks in front of strangers — *'in public trying to open my wallet and several everyday tasks when you go out'* — also created anxiety.

Almost two-thirds of respondents (n=101) indicated that they experienced depression as a result of their lymphoedema. Difficulty in accepting the lymphoedema was identified by many as the main cause of their depression. Several comments such as the following were made: *'I accepted the mastectomy but I cannot accept the lymphoedema'*, and, *'I just want to state that suffering from lymphoedema daily is harder for me than having my breast off, chemotherapy or radiotherapy. I think that the worst thing is forever, and everyone knows and sees it'*. The realisation that they had been inflicted with a condition which they perceived as *'a life sentence of disability'*, and the need to come to terms with the *'foreverness'* of the situation contributed to the depression experienced by several respondents.

## Access to management of the lymphoedema

Inability to gain assistance from the health care system made people feel abandoned. Many commented that their fears, concerns, and difficulties, incurred as a result of living with lymphoedema, had been trivialised by health professionals, with comments such as *'Oh, people make too much of lymphoedema'*. Several other comments such as *'When the problem [lymphoedema] started the surgeon showed me the door and said, "Go and see your GP"'* were made. It was also reported that, in most instances, general practitioners do not know how to seek assistance for the management of the lymphoedema.

When the respondents were correctly informed as how to access treatment, the cost of regular treatment, which is mostly available through the private health care system, was prohibitive for many. As one woman commented '. . . *cost of trying to live a pain- and debilitation-free life. I have just had 12 weeks of two to three lymphoedema treatments per week costing me $3200 so far. Nothing back from MBF'*. Many of those who had had the size of the limb reduced through the use of complex physical therapy found that they needed regular treatments to maintain the limb at a reasonable size. Many funds do not reimburse even part of the cost of therapist treatment or reimburse any of the cost of compression garments which are the mainstay of management as their use prevents the limb from becoming more swollen. These garments can cost up to $600 each and last for only three to four months, and at least two garments are needed at any one time. The cost, plus the lack of information made available on how to manage their lymphoedema, left many feeling powerless to take control of their lives.

# DISCUSSION

It is very clear from the findings of this study that individuals have complex physical and psychological health care needs as a consequence of their lymphoedema. Physically many respondents had been ignored and this had a direct impact on their quality of life through impairing their ability to mobilise, to socialise and, in some instances, to participate in employment. Emotional issues and lifestyle changes that people endure as a result of this life sentence of disability were, for some, totally devastating. These problems are compounded when fears, concerns and difficulties are trivialised by health professionals. Further to this, the inability to access assistance for the management of the lymphoedema from the health care system left many with the feeling of being abandoned.

The findings from this study emphasise the need for health professionals to incorporate a holistic approach when caring for individuals with lymphoedema. To be fully effective attention must be given not only to the oedematous limb or body part, but also to the physical and psychological perceptions of each patient. Access to health care for the management of lymphoedema also needs to become more available.

# References

Badger C (1987): Lymphoedema: Management of patients with advanced cancer. *The Professional Nurse* January: 100–102.

Casley-Smith Judith (1992): Modern treatment of lymphoedema. *Modern Medicine* 35 5, May: 70–83.

Collard V (1990): Understanding lymphoedema and the occupational therapist's role. *The Australian Occupational Therapy Journal* 37 2, June: 109–111.

Consensus Document of the International Society of Lymphology Executive Committee (1995): The diagnosis and treatment of peripheral oedema. *Lymphology* 28: 113–117.

Foldi E, Foldi M, Weissleder H (1985): Conservative treatment of lymphoedema of the limbs. *Angiology* 36 3, March: 171–180.

Foldi M (1985): Complex decongestive therapy. *Progress in Lymphology, X. Proceedings of the Xth International Congress of Lymphology.* Adelaide: University of Adelaide Press. pp. 165–167.

Granda C (1994): Nursing management of patients with lymphoedema associated with breast cancer therapy. *Cancer Nursing* 17 3: 229–235.

Gray B (1987): Management of limb oedema in advanced cancer. *Nursing Times* 9 December, 83 9: 39–40.

Humble C (1995): Lymphoedema: Incidence, pathophysiology, management, and nursing care. *Oncology Nursing Forum* 22 10:1503–1509.

Williams A (1997): Update: Lymphoedema. *Professional Nurse* 12 9, June: 645–648.

# Research piece B

## *Breast cancer diagnosis — detection methods and emotions*

*Linda Reaby*

Breast cancer is a treatable disease that can be cured if detected in the early stages. Currently a combination of breast self-examination (BSE), appropriate clinical examination and mammograph screening are the recommended methods for early breast cancer detection (Stager, 1993).

A study by Nettles-Carlson (1989) showed that only 18–34 per cent of women practise monthly BSE. Breast tumours found by touch, either by accident or during BSE, tend to be larger — generally, at least 15 mm in diameter — than those found by mammography (Townsend, 1987). More than 60 per cent of carcinomas detected by mammography screening in Australia are impalpable and thus would have been missed on BSE and clinical examination (Rickard et al., 1991). However, there are a number of women who are not taking advantage of mammography screening programs. For example, in a survey of women aged 40–75, Schechter et al. (1990) found that respondents associated breast cancer primarily with mastectomy and death and cited fear of discovering they might have the disease as a reason for not having mammograms. When women comprehend that early detection is possible their fear of the disease could be greatly reduced.

My study addressed the issues of breast problem detection, investigation of the problem, and emotions experienced when the diagnosis of breast cancer is confirmed. Its purpose was to determine:

1.  how a group of 95 women initially detected their breast problems;

2.  if they had their breast problems investigated immediately or had delayed diagnosis; and

3.  what initial fears and feelings these women experienced when diagnosed with breast cancer.

Letters were sent to a total of 188 female patients. Of these, 95 women consented to participate in the study — a 50.5 per cent response rate. An interview schedule was designed to assist in answering the study's questions. It consisted predominantly of open-ended questions that were arranged in the order in which the women's experiences would most likely have occurred so as to aid recall.

A majority of women were married (64%), white Australian (73%), protestant (58%), had completed secondary schooling (59%), had private health insurance (76%), claimed to have a very good to excellent chance for a cure (65%), and required no post-mastectomy radiation (86%) or chemotherapy (72%). The mean age for the population was 56.25 years. There were 44 women (46%) who were 55 years of age or younger.

## HOW THE WOMEN FOUND THEIR BREAST CANCER

The women were asked to describe how their breast cancer was initially discovered. This is shown in Table B.1. Twenty-nine women detected a breast lump by chance (usually in the shower). BSE revealed a breast lump in 23 women. Eighteen women noticed another indicator — nipple discharge, soreness in the breast, inverted nipple, rash/itchy nipple, swollen arm and hand, thickening of the skin around the breast, and dimpling of the breast. For 10 women a doctor's physical examination gave the first indication that a breast problem existed — the examination either revealed a palpable lump or aroused the physician's suspicion of cancer. A mammogram was the first indicator of a potential problem for 15 women.

The vast majority of the women experienced myriad negative emotional feelings when a lump was detected.

*I was watching television and I put my hand on my breast and I felt this hard lump. I started to cry. I thought it was the end of my life. I just knew that it was cancer. My mother had breast cancer when she was in her early 50s so I had started to check my breasts every month since turning 40. When I felt that lump I knew my nightmare had come true. I started to scream and shake because I was so frightened. It was terrible.*

Regular BSE was not practised by 41 women. The following are interview excerpts of two women stating their reasons for not performing BSE:

*I never had the courage to test my breasts for lumps. You hear all these horrible stories about women who get breast cancer and everything that they have to go through and they die anyway. I immediately thought about these things when I was diagnosed and it was so upsetting and devastating.*

*I have known too many women who have died horrific deaths because of breast cancer. I just could never bring myself to examine my breast. I was so petrified that I might find something and I just didn't want to have to face that. It's a silly mentality but that was how I coped. I was just lucky that I found the lump just by chance when I was showering, but when I did I just went crazy with fear.*

**Table B.1. Initial methods of breast cancer detection**

| Methods | Breast cancer group (N=95) | |
| --- | --- | --- |
| | n | % |
| By chance | 29 | 30 |
| Breast self-examination | 23 | 24 |
| Visible symptoms | 18 | 19 |
| Mammography | 15 | 16 |
| Clinical examination | 10 | 11 |

Seventy-three women had their lumps, symptoms or suspicious findings evaluated when they consulted medical practitioners. They were immediately referred for tests that proved positive for breast cancer. Twenty-two women had delayed diagnosis of breast cancer two weeks to eight months.

Ten women who delayed having their breast symptoms investigated gave a variety of reasons for their procrastination. The fear of mastectomy was the primary deterrent to early presentation by some of these women.

*I had a mammogram because my friend was having one. They detected something and suggested that I should have it seen to or removed. I didn't because I was so scared of the idea of having surgery and losing my breast. Six months later I could feel a lump under the nipple. I went to a specialist who did a biopsy and it was cancerous. I was really shocked, I didn't think it was possible.*

There were other women whose mothers, grandmothers and/or aunts had had a mastectomy. These women's memories of their relatives' experiences compounded their fears and caused them to delay investigation of breast symptoms.

*I woke up and found blood in the bed but there wasn't any lump. At the time my daughter was getting married and I was very busy with the wedding and I ignored it. It progressively got worse and I decided that I'd cut myself. One day I found blood in my bra. I knew it must have been coming from the nipple, and I pressed the nipple and blood came out. I had a feeling it was something serious but I couldn't deal with it then so I waited three weeks until after my daughter was married and on her honeymoon before I went to the doctor. I went for a mammogram and that evening the doctor told me straight away that it was definitely cancer. I was terrified because I had seen my mother's sister go through so much because she had breast cancer and a mastectomy and I just couldn't deal with it.*

Several women had seen their friends experience the physical and psychological pain of the disease.

*I discovered a lump in the shower. I was also losing weight. I decided to do nothing about it because I had seen a couple of my friends battle with chemotherapy. They were living unbelievably dreadful lives and that wasn't for me. About eight months later . . . my husband talked me into seeing a surgeon who did a biopsy that showed cancer. I delayed having the mastectomy done . . . I didn't think I was going to survive it mentally or physically.*

A few women observed both good and poor health management of their loved ones and there were others who had seen the disease progress and cause death.

*I was having a shower and I found there was a lump. I had nursed so many women who had breast cancer and many of them died such painful deaths. I thought the same thing was going to happen to me so I went on a three-week holiday and then saw the doctor two weeks after I returned. It took me that long to get up the nerve and confidence to see someone about it.*

Other women had distorted images about breast cancer — mental images of pain, dependency issues, ugliness, life struggles and fears about dying.

*I didn't feel a lump but I knew my breast didn't look right. I was so frightened that it was cancer and that I would have to go through all that awful treatment, be cut up and scarred, lose my hair, waste away and die a slow and painful death. I waited for about six months and when I went for my pap smear the doctor checked my breast and sent me for a mammogram. I had a biopsy that confirmed it was cancer and my whole world fell apart.*

Twelve women had delayed diagnosis due primarily to lack of physical examination and inadequate investigation of pertinent family history by medical practitioners.

*I might get a bit teary telling you about this, it was terrible. I was four months pregnant and I had a lump in my left breast and the doctor just presumed that it was a blocked duct. He didn't do any examination of the lump at all. I asked him about it several times during the next several months but he just acted like I was being neurotic about the whole thing. Once I started to lactate the lump got huge so I became really concerned and went to my GP and he immediately referred me to a surgeon who did a biopsy.*

There were women in this group who felt that the physicians were not listening to them.

*I went to a doctor and she was concerned because my breasts were so lumpy and she couldn't examine them properly so she sent me for a mammogram that found cysts in my right breast. The radiologist at the breast clinic recommended that I have mammograms more often because of my lumpy breasts.*

*Unfortunately, my regular doctor got very sick and stopped practising. I told the doctor who took her place my story but she told me that all that was silly and for me not to worry because I was too young for breast cancer. This went on for several years, I was feeling really tired. She checked my breasts and I asked her if I could have a mammogram because I couldn't get one without a referral. She said 'No, no, no' and 'How old are you?' I told her I was 43 and she said 'Just let it go.' About five months later I felt a bit of a lump and because my breasts were lumpy anyway I thought 'I'll let it go'. It was still there two months later. Fortunately, my regular doctor was away and the other doctor who saw me gave me a referral to the breast clinic. When I did go they immediately diagnosed it as breast cancer. If only the doctor would have listened to me. It was a very hard time in my life.*

Some of these women felt that the medical practitioners gave false reassurances to them when they presented with their breast complaints or concerns.

*I found that I had a lump in the left upper quadrant of my left breast and I immediately made an appointment. I went to my GP and he gave me an external examination. He said that it was nonmalignant but he could define the edges of the tumour and it felt cystic rather than malignant and not to worry but to come back in four months and to take Oil of Evening Primrose to help calm me down. In that four months the lump just got bigger and bigger and when I went back I had an immediate biopsy.*

## HOW THE WOMEN FELT

**Table B.2 Feelings when diagnosed with breast cancer**

| Feelings | Breast cancer group (N=93) (Responses n=168) | |
|---|---|---|
| | n | % |
| Stunned/shocked | 59 | 35 |
| Devastation | 34 | 21 |
| Resignation | 13 | 8 |
| Unfair/why me | 11 | 7 |
| Anger | 10 | 6 |
| Guilt | 8 | 5 |
| Concern for family | 7 | 4 |
| Get rid of it | 6 | 3 |
| Get on with life | 6 | 3 |
| Denial | 4 | 2 |
| Panic | 4 | 2 |
| Loneliness | 3 | 2 |
| Optimistic | 2 | 1 |
| Expected it | 1 | 1 |

The women were asked to remember how they felt when they were first told by their doctor that they had breast cancer. Two women reported that they had no initial feelings but 93 women reported 168 feelings ranging from devastation to optimism (see Table B.2).

*I felt utterly devastated and utterly horrified. I had never expected it. It was very hard for me to accept and I cried continuously for a week. I thought I would never be the same.*

## WHAT WOMEN FEARED ABOUT DIAGNOSIS

The women were asked what fears they experienced when told of their breast cancer diagnosis. The predominant fears were: dying from the disease, spreading of the cancer and leaving loved ones.

*To me it was like a death sentence because at that stage I knew that I had this darn thing for at least 12 to 15 months. This had to be an advanced cancer and that really devastated me. I was positive that it would go all through my body. It is still in the back of my mind.*

Other fears mentioned less often were: losing the affected breast, experiencing pain, having chemotherapy, incurring a financial burden due to treatment of the disease, having residual physical limitations, having to be hospitalised, receiving an anaesthetic, and being alone.

**Table B.3 Fears when diagnosed with breast cancer**

| Fears | n | Breast cancer group (N=95) (Responses n=121) % |
|---|---|---|
| Dying | 45 | 37 |
| Cancer spreading | 22 | 18 |
| Leaving loved ones | 18 | 15 |
| Losing the breast | 12 | 10 |
| Pain | 9 | 7 |
| Chemotherapy | 7 | 5 |
| Physical limitations | 3 | 3 |
| Costs of treatments | 2 | 2 |
| Hospitalisation | 1 | 1 |
| Anaesthetic | 1 | 1 |
| Being alone | 1 | 1 |

My study confirms the findings of Nettles-Carlson (1989) that only 18–34 per cent of women practise BSE. Only 24 per cent of women in my study practised BSE. The literature shows that two major barriers to BSE are the fear of finding a lump and the fear of breast cancer (Nettles-Carlson, 1989). I also found these barriers in my study.

The statements made by my study's participants during the interviews indicate the terror and the crisis they experienced when they first detected a breast lump or suspected that something was wrong. During this stressful period, therapeutic intervention is required. This intervention is generally sought from a variety of health professionals. Their major role should involve assisting the woman in obtaining appropriate medical evaluation; dealing with the impact that the detection of a lump has upon one's life; being cognisant of the possible ramifications of a mastectomy; and utilising appropriate support systems for the woman's benefit. These pre-diagnostic services are not routinely offered. Instituting these services would decrease women's anxiety and help them to deal more effectively with the potential health threat.

About 10 per cent of Australian women with breast symptoms neglect them and delay having them investigated (Women's Health Issues, 1989). The same percentage occurred in my study.

Researchers have documented that women harbour many misconceptions about breast cancer that lead to fear, panic and avoidance (Felzer, 1988; Schechter et al., 1990). Similar misconceptions were also found in my study. Health professionals need to take these misconceptions into consideration as playing a part in women's reactions to the disease. Some women experience such profound fear and panic that they delay medical attention to suspicious breast problems for weeks and even months. The commonly cited causes of delay by women in having a breast problem investigated are ignorance, fear of the diagnosis of cancer, fear of disfigurement from mastectomy, fear of hospitals in general and surgery in particular, and a fatalistic attitude (Felzer, 1988). As indicated by the interview excerpts presented in this paper, the women's fear of and anxiety at being diagnosed with breast cancer contributed to their delaying investigation The possible health threat of breast cancer evoked a sense of crisis in the women that hampered their abilities to make competent decisions about definitive investigation of the symptoms.

Over 50 per cent of the women in my study who had delayed diagnosis due to inadequate medical investigation were under the age of 50. Although breast cancer generally occurs less frequently in younger women, in 1992, of the 7000 women diagnosed with breast cancer in Australia, 2000 were under the age of 50 (Conry, 1994). This statistic clearly indicates that a large number of younger women are being diagnosed with the disease each year. Therefore, when younger women present to their medical practitioner with a breast complaint, they require a thorough assessment of the problem. Women should also be encouraged to seek additional medical opinions if they have doubts about the thoroughness of their breast problem investigation.

Many women who delay seeking a medical opinion will feel guilt and many women who have delays due to medical mismanagement will experience anger. These women need avenues to express these feelings, which should be accepted calmly by all caregivers. Such sympathetic acceptance could both allay the guilt and anger of the moment and establish the foundation of relationships continuing throughout treatment. Therapeutic relationships decrease the stress and crisis that women experience and enhance their abilities to take control of their lives through competent decision-making about breast cancer treatments. In addition, it is crucial to find ways to help women to seek advice early so that more treatment options can be made available to them, and so that their survival time can be lengthened.

A diagnosis of breast cancer is an experience that no woman ever wants to confront. The treatment of cancer is seen in most people not merely as a current physical injury or threat of physical death but equally strongly as an emotional catastrophe.

Formal education programs need to be implemented. They should focus on reducing women's fears of breast cancer and increasing knowledge about breast cancer and its detection. The major points to be stressed during these programs are that women need to monitor their breast cancer status and that early detection can mean cure in 90 per cent of cases (J. Forbes, personal communication, 12 June 1997).

The results also show that there is a need for a specific health professional to assist women newly diagnosed with breast cancer. This individual would assume several roles, including one of advocacy and support for the women, and ensuring that they have correct and needed information regarding their disease. Registered nurse oncology specialists have the medical, psychological, and sociological knowledge to deal with women newly diagnosed with breast cancer. The attention, understanding and support of a knowledgeable, competent oncology nurse specialist is as essential as the effective treatment for control of the disease.

Nurses also need to be involved in community health breast education programs, organising health festivals, developing and disseminating materials on breast cancer prevention and detection, providing public lectures on the disease, and designing programs for community education and the mass media.

The only means at present to reduce the morbidity and mortality of the disease is through early detection, and education is the key to achieving this goal.

## Acknowledgments

This study was part of a larger project supported by a Human Services and Health Research and Development Grant from the Commonwealth Department of Human Services and Health, and a research grant from the University of Canberra.

## References

Collins J (1994): The role of the surgeon. *Cancer Forum* 18: 92–95.

Commonwealth Department of Health, Housing and Community Services, Working Party of the National Advisory Committee for the Early Detection of Breast Cancer (1992): National program for the early detection of breast cancer. *National Accreditation Guidelines, 21 November 1991.* Canberra: Australian Government Publishing Service.

Conry C (1994): Evaluation of a breast complaint: Is it cancer? *American Family Physician* 49: 445–450.

Felzer SG (1988): *The Psychosocial Impact of Breast Cancer and Its Treatment.* Ann Arbor: UMI Dissertation Information Service.

Lee-Feldstein A, Anton-Culver H, Feldstein PJ (1994): Treatment differences and other prognostic factors related to breast cancer survival. *JAMA* 271: 1163–1168.

National Health and Medical Research Council (1995): *Clinical Practice Guidelines: The Management of Early Breast Cancer.* Canberra: Australian Government Publishing Service.

Neilsen B, East D (1990): Advances in breast cancer. *Nursing Clinics of North America* 25: 365–375.

Nettles-Carlson B (1989): Early detection of breast cancer. *Journal of Obstetrics, Gynaecology and Neonatal Nursing* 18: 373–381.

Rickard MT, Lee W, Read JW (1991): Breast cancer diagnosis by screening mammography: Early results of the Central Sydney Area Health Service Breast X-ray Programme. *Medical Journal of Australia* 154: 126–131.

Schechter C, Vanchieri CF, Crofton C (1990): Evaluating women's attitudes and perceptions in developing mammography promotion messages. *Public Health Report* 105: 253–257.

Townsend CM (1987): Management of breast cancer: Surgery and adjuvant therapy. *Clinical Symposia* 39: 3–32.

Women's Health Issues — Breast Health (1989): Australia's mastectomy rates are too high. *Australian Medicine* 1, November: 426.

Stager JL (1993): The comprehensive breast cancer knowledge test: Validity and reliability. *Journal of Advanced Nursing* 18: 1133–1140.

## Personal communication

J. Forbes, 12 June 1997

# Research piece C

## Adcare Lifestyle Retreat — empowerment and enrichment for people living with cancer

*Ann Fowler, Gloria Swift, Lucia Apolloni*

## PREAMBLE

The Adcare Lifestyle Retreat is the brainchild of Gloria Swift, Oncology Nurse Consultant at Warilla Community Health Centre in New South Wales, Australia. Gloria saw in her clients a need to change their lifestyle to incorporate healthy diet, exercise, relaxation, fun and support systems. She conceived the idea of a five-day retreat for people living with cancer. Her energy, enthusiasm and phenomenal organising ability got the first retreat off the ground. Ann Fowler first became involved when Gloria asked her to present a stress management workshop at the 1996 retreat. As Clinical Nurse Consultant Quality Management at the Illawarra Health Service in New South Wales, Ann saw a great opportunity to evaluate the positive outcomes she had witnessed anecdotally. Lucia Apolloni became involved in the development of a tool of evaluation and the collation of results. In 1997 it was decided to use a validated tool to measure before and after effects. The results are presented in this paper.

## INTRODUCTION

Literature indicates that exposure to stress, or stressful events, can be a powerful contributor to illness (King et al., 1987). In addition, loneliness or lack of support for people with cancer exacerbates the risk of recurrence of the disease (Lambley, 1987). People living with cancer and their carers have a high incidence of stress-related conditions. Constant emotional and physical demands on a day-to-day basis can lower the immune system and increase vulnerability to cancer (Lambley et al. 1987; King, 1987; Munro, 1992; Klarreich, 1988). Hans Selye (1976) defined stress as 'the non-specific response of the body to any demand made on it', while William Wilkie (1995:8) referred to negative stress as being a 'significant impairment of function, resulting from excessive load on the nervous system'. Herbert Benson (1975) stated that 'environmental demands require behavioural adjustment' and maintained that physical changes such as brain wave frequency, decreased blood pressure, decreased blood lactate and a decrease in muscle tension are a consequence of relaxation, which counteracts the effects of negative stress.

# BACKGROUND

In 1993 our close interaction with people living with cancer revealed a need for adults with cancer and their carers to participate actively in managing their own quality of life. They also needed respite care, support systems and empowerment. After reference to literature (see above), we hypothesised that relaxation practices, natural therapies and the correct use of support groups, if taught to clients and carers living with cancer, could reduce the risk of recurrence of the disease, increase remission periods, reduce the risk of carers' incidence of illness and enable clients and carers to actively maintain their own wellness. The literature also suggested that by adopting the abovementioned strategies there was also the possibility of reducing the risk of incidence of illness in surviving relatives/partners after a death. In order to address the perceived needs of adults living with cancer a five-day retreat for clients and carers was conceived. The first adult care (Adcare) retreat was organised in 1994.

Support for the planning and implementation of the retreat was obtained from area health service management and field workers. A program was developed that included activities, entertainment, workshops in lifestyle management and education. The retreat concept, as well as giving respite care, offered an opportunity for people to network and become acquainted with support groups.

Because of the success of the initial retreat and requests for the idea to continue, the Adcare Lifestyle Retreat has become an annual event. Breast Cancer Support Group members who have been to earlier retreats have become volunteers at the retreat house, helping with housekeeping duties as well as participating in the activities.

# PROJECT

The Adcare Lifestyle Retreats considered in this exploratory study were conducted at Stanwell Tops Christian Conference Centre in New South Wales for five days each in March 1996 and April 1997. They included workshops on lifestyle issues, stress management, complementary therapies, herbal remedies, meditation/relaxation techniques and practices, tai chi, therapeutic and aromatherapy massage, naturopathic consultations, reiki, craft, gentle exercise, walks, swimming, aquarobics and entertainment. Two important components of both retreats were laughter and responsibility. Each person was part of a team responsible on rotation for domestic duties such as table setting and washing up. The highlight of each retreat was the concert. Teams were given limited resources but they produced theatrical events of remarkably high quality and enjoyment.

# METHOD

Longitudinal evaluations were conducted to ascertain the effect of relaxation techniques, stress management workshops, participation in support groups, exercise and alternative therapies. After each retreat a follow-up study was conducted to evaluate the long-term effects — whether the concepts presented in the retreat were taken up and practised and what benefit this practice had on the participants' perception of their general wellbeing. Because of factors such as deaths and movements away from the district, before, after and telephone responses do not always refer to the same number of respondents so the percentages are not statistically comparable but the statistics quoted for the surveys give a clear indication of the trends within the group of respondents.

## The participants

The participants were people who had been diagnosed with cancer, carers of people with cancer and people who were in remission. In 1996 39 people attended, 59 per cent for the first time. In 1997 49 people attended and 36.7 per cent were first-time attendees.

## Evaluation

In 1996 a locally constructed questionnaire was distributed before the retreat and at the end of the retreat and a follow-up telephone interview was conducted six months later. In 1997 a General Health Questionnaire (GHQ12) (Goldberg, 1978) was issued prior to the retreat. A copy of the questions is contained in Figure C.1. Questions were also asked on relaxation practice and support group attendance. A follow-up telephone interview using the same questions was conducted four months after the retreat.

In 1996, 34 participants completed the questionnaire at the retreat. Of these, 26 completed the questionnaire again when telephoned. In 1997 34 participants completed the questionnaire before the retreat and 29 completed the questionnaire again when telephoned.

# RESULTS

Overall there was an improvement in the general wellbeing of respondents in the longitudinal study of both retreats. The results of the 1997 GHQ12 (Goldberg, 1978) indicated a level of improvement on every item of the scale for the group of respondents.

**Figure C.1 Questions asked of Adcare participants involved in the 1997 retreat**

The following 12 questions are from the General Health Questionnaire (GHQ12) (Goldberg, 1978).

Have you, over the past few weeks:

- been able to concentrate on whatever you're doing?

- lost much sleep over worry?

- felt that you are playing a useful part in thing?

- felt capable of making decisions about things?

- felt constantly under strain?

- felt that you couldn't overcome your difficulties?

- been able to enjoy your normal day-to-day activities?

- been able to face up to your problems?

- been feeling unhappy and depressed?

- been losing confidence in yourself?

- been thinking of yourself as a worthless person?

- been feeling reasonably happy all things considered?

In 1996, 97 per cent of the 26 respondents stated that the Adcare Lifestyle Retreat had helped them become more aware of the factors in their life that cause stress. In 1997, among the 29 telephone respondents, there was an increase of 32 per cent in the frequency of weekly and daily practice of relaxation. In 1996 results indicated that, after a period of six months, relaxation practice on a regular basis had increased by 17 per cent — 74 per cent of the 26 people who answered the follow-up telephone questionnaire were practising relaxation daily (27 per cent) and weekly (47 per cent). Of those who practised regular relaxation techniques 95 per cent said the information given at the retreat regarding these techniques was useful. 19 per cent of the 26 respondents said they could not do relaxation before the retreat. One respondent remarked that *relaxation is keeping me sane*. Types of relaxation and stress-relieving techniques practised were yoga, tai chi, breathing, massage, relaxation with music, and meditation/visualisation tapes and classes.

In interviews with 26 respondents six months after the 1996 retreat 42 per cent talked of the support network that the retreat had created and the importance of this network. One person whose partner had died remarked that *the system of people who went to the retreat supported [partner], and I now use that support system for myself*. Another participant, referring to her need for support, said *I couldn't do it on my own*.

Before the 1996 retreat, 59 per cent of those who filled out the questionnaire participated in a cancer support group. Six months after the retreat, 58 per cent of the 26 who responded to the follow-up telephone questionnaire were attending a cancer support group but a further 35 per cent of the 26 were attending a craft group which they considered to be a support group.

In 1997 the attendance at support groups among the 29 interviewed by telephone increased by only 3 per cent, from 76 per cent to 79 per cent. This could be due to the fact that the retreat was advertised through cancer support groups so the participants were drawn from this population.

Six months after the 1996 retreat 62 per cent of the 26 who responded to the follow-up telephone questionnaire were using natural therapies such as naturopathy and herbal remedies; 87 per cent of the 26 said they had found the information given at the retreat very useful. In the 1997 group of 29 telephone respondents the practice of natural healing methods also increased markedly.

In 1996 the proportion of participants rating their emotional state as 'good' or 'great' prior to the retreat was 39 per cent. At the end of the retreat 94 per cent of the 34 rated their emotional state as 'good' or 'great'. Six months after the retreat 61 per cent of the 26 who responded to the follow-up telephone questionnaire reported that they were emotionally good or very good.

Prior to the 1996 retreat a total of 45 per cent of the 34 participants had reported their physical wellbeing as good or very good. At the end of the retreat 90 per cent of the 34 responded that they felt good or very good. Six months after the retreat 50 per cent of the 26 who responded to the follow-up telephone questionnaire reported feeling very good and 27 per cent of the 26 were feeling good, a total of 77 per cent.

## DISCUSSION

Peter Lambley in *The Psychology of Cancer* (1987:63) states that 'people who experience anxiety and stress on a routine day-to-day level tend to have persistently lower natural killer cell activity (NKCA) measures than people who don't experience high levels of anxiety', while Munro (1992:42) says 'stress and immunity are interconnected'. Herbert Benson in *The Relaxation Response* (1975) suggests that regular relaxation counteracts the psychological and physical harm incurred by poor coping and negative stress. This literature suggests that stress reduction in clients with cancer will reduce the incidence of recurrence of disease and increase remission periods. Stress reduction in carers of people with cancer may reduce their risk of disease/illness. The exposure to stress or stressful demands can be a powerful contributing factor in physical disorders (King, 1987).

In light of this the findings of the exploratory studies of the Adcare Lifestyle Retreat carried out in 1996 and 1997 indicate a positive response, with an increase in regular practice of relaxation for both samples (17 per cent of the 26 telephone respondents in 1996 and 32 per cent of the 29 respondents in 1997). Comments made by respondents indicate that 15 per cent of the 1996 telephone respondents experienced changes in lifestyle and attitudes, and increased happiness. One respondent commented that she had *'never been so relaxed'*. This is significant in light of the indication that

> poor coping and stress lowers the immune system and this over time can create a chronic vulnerability to growths (Lambley, 1987:63).

Lambley (1987) goes on to say that

> forming a workable personal relationship, all other factors being equal, is the key to survival.

Though the 1996 figures for telephone respondents revealed a 1 per cent fall in the number of people who reported attending a cancer support group, 35 per cent attended a craft group which they saw as a support group. Some respondents said they did not do much (or any) craft but saw the group purely as a support system. Some of this number also attended more than one group. In their comments 42 per cent of the telephone respondents mentioned the importance of support networking and how the retreat initiated that for them.

By educating people living with cancer in many different aspects of healthy lifestyle the Adcare Lifestyle Retreat has empowered consumers to be in control of their own wellness. The retreat process has facilitated the promotion of health awareness, the prevention of illness and growth of responsibility for self. It has been instrumental in encouraging and enabling participants to accept and maintain control in their lifestyle choices. Morgan (1990) emphasises that self-care empowers the consumer.

Overall the Adcare Lifestyle Retreat has proved to be of great benefit not only to clients with cancer but also to their carers and those who have lost a relative to cancer within the last two years. Comments such as *'a great concept'* and *'a new beginning'* illustrate the achievement of improved outcomes as a result of the project. This is an innovative program which has achieved its aim to improve and effectively make changes to the quality of the lives of people living with cancer and is best illustrated in the comments made by one participant, Janet Jones:

*I was most apprehensive about coming as I knew no-one but within minutes felt so very welcome. The energy and support and love of this retreat was something I have never experienced before. Before this week, with my treatment, time in hospital etc. I really felt that my life was out of control. This week has given me time to step back from everything, experience a range of ideas and therapies. I now feel in charge again, know what therapies*

*I want to begin and feel much more positive and ready to get on with my life. Thank you so much.*

Janet died in August 1997.

**Further information about this project can be obtained from Gloria Swift, Oncology Nurse Consultant, Warilla Community Health Centre, Belfast Avenue, Warilla, New South Wales 2528, Australia. Telephone +61-2-4296-4200.**

**For information concerning the evaluation of the retreats, contact Ann Fowler, Clinical Nurse Consultant (Quality), Illawarra Community Health Service, PO Box 238, Warilla, New South Wales 2528, Australia. Telephone +61-2-4229-2755.**

## Acknowledgment

We thank Janet Jones's husband and family for allowing us to use the comment she made on her evaluation of the Adcare Lifestyle Retreat.

## References

Benson H (1975): *The Relaxation Response*. New York: William Morrow & Co.

Goldberg DP (1978): *Manual of General Health Questionnaire*. Windsor: Nfer-Nelson.

Klarreich SH (1988): *The Stress Solution — A Rational Approach to Increasing Corporate and Personal Effectiveness*. Toronto, Canada: Key Porter Books Ltd.

King M, Stanley G, Burrows G (1987): *Stress Theory and Practice*. Australia: Grune & Stratton.

Lambley P (1987): *The Psychology of Cancer*. London: Macdonald & Co.

Morgan A (1990): Health teaching in clinical nursing practice. *The Australian Journal of Advanced Nursing* 17 4: 37–40.

Munro KI (1992): CRF Regulation and Integration of Pituitary-adrenal and Central Nervous System Responses to Stress. In: Pfister HP (ed.): *Stress Effects on Central and Peripheral System*. Queensland: Australian Academic Press Pty Ltd, pp. 39–50.

Selye H (1976): *The Stress of Life*. New York: McGraw-Hill.

Wilkie W (1995): *Understanding Stress Breakdown*. Alexandria, NSW: EJ Dwyer.

# Research piece D

## What CanTeen members think about their treatment

*Anthony Cammell*

## PREAMBLE

CanTeen is the shorthand but well-known name for the Australian Teenage Cancer Patients' Society Ltd. Anthony Cammell has been State Coordinator of CanTeen in South Australia since 1995. He has written this paper to, in his own words, *'educate' nursing staff of our members' thoughts regarding their hospital experiences. I have regular contact with these young people living with cancer and I often hear their comments on treatment and their time in hospital.*

## BACKGROUND

CanTeen members were asked to comment on a number of broad questions about:

- provision of care as both inpatient and outpatient;
- communication from medical staff; and
- scope or extent of care outside strict medical boundaries.

The young people were given guidelines but were provided also with freedom to comment on whatever they deemed relevant. The value in accessing these young people is in having the experience, perceptions and feedback not just of the patients but also of their siblings, and all this information is recent and very relevant to nurses. The feedback is from hospitals around Australia and therefore provides an overall reflection of medical practices Australia wide. Interestingly patients who were treated four or more years ago commented on aspects of care that were not mentioned by more recently treated patients. It seems that, in conjunction with advances in treatment regimes, there have also been great strides in psychological care, not only for the patient, but for siblings and parents too.

## CARE WHILE AN INPATIENT

Most of our members realise that oncology is a very difficult and demanding area for all involved and generally everyone is doing their best to make the stay in hospital as pleasant and pain free as possible.

A lot of adjectives were used in comments under this heading: *'very good'*, *'professional'*, *'excellent'*, and *'supportive'* all kept appearing, and are a credit to the staff involved. Members recognised and praised personal and informed care and they appreciated being treated as adults, with staff taking an interest in their progress and how they were coping. These efforts by staff lessened the trauma of the hospital stay. Where these facets of care were absent, the time in hospital was perceived as much more stressful. Our members generally acknowledged that staff made every effort for the patients' comfort, and that this care was evident from the first day of treatment to the last.

Members also suggested opportunities for improvement, and a number of themes were repeated throughout the country. Obviously, for practical reasons, a number of these changes and rearrangements may be unworkable at any given time. The purpose of mentioning them is simply to reinforce their importance and to acknowledge them.

## Suggested improvements

A number of patients were uncomfortable about being placed with children much younger than themselves. Those who mentioned this expressed dislike for sharing space with someone below their development and maturity. This is a typical adolescent reaction but it raises issues of total care, and the benefits of being able to share experiences and empathise with another in the same situation. Many members cited the advantages of not being *'alone'* with their treatment and that being placed with, or having access to, young people of a similar age made a big difference to their hospital experience. One member who was placed with children for a short time noticed that the staff were coming to her for conversation and time out from the youngsters! Another member commented that the nurses were accessing him for *'time outs'* from the elderly.

There were the expected complaints of boredom, pain, grim surroundings and isolation. These were not presented as being necessarily solvable or a nursing responsibility, but as facts of hospitalisation. It was also apparent that there have been large improvements in these areas in the last few years.

It was suggested that involving parents and siblings with the treatment wherever possible or appropriate made a difference to how connected the family unit felt.

Of course this is a highly subjective area. Not every family wants a large degree of involvement, and washing and personal care would be the last thing that a lot of adolescents would want from their parents. The principal area of improvement was the involvement of siblings in the progress of the treatment and ensuring that everyone in the family who wanted to be was aware and informed. Although this is a tough one it was mentioned enough times to warrant nursing staff being aware of it and, when possible, being flexible for each family.

Interestingly the bulk of the suggestions for changes came under the areas of psychological care and family inclusion. In this age of increased professional responsibility and multiskilling it would seem that more and more of the previously outsourced tasks are being expected of the nursing staff. Not only are they the primary caregivers in the wards but they are now being expected to be sensitive to and responsible for the state of mind of parents and siblings as well as of patients.

# COMMUNICATION AND INFORMATION TRANSFER

A number of members said that their parents were kept informed about what was going on but that they themselves had only a bare grasp of their treatment and very little idea of where it was going. The one commonality amongst those surveyed was, perhaps, their hesitancy to ask questions. The problem would be alleviated if nursing staff could explain as they went along, and doctors and specialists could make sure that things are broadly understood by the patient, not just by the parents.

Some members spoke of first conferences between the parents and the doctor, with a second conference including the patient. Examples of this came from members as young as 14 and as old as 17. They expressed a sense of isolation, and some suspicion of what they were not being told. They said that this felt threatening. This is especially significant given the already vulnerable position they were in. Coupled with this is the recurring mention of *'blank spots'* immediately after being told of the diagnosis. This generally meant that a lot of the positive information that was relayed in that first meeting was lost to the patient. If patients were not confident about asking questions or simply didn't think to ask the right questions, then information might not be relayed for some time.

Related to this is the issue of siblings often being left out. Due to understandable pressures, parents do not necessarily include siblings in conversations once treatment has begun, and not everyone thinks to include them in the initial conferences that explain what is going to happen over the ensuing months. This oversight often results in siblings distancing themselves and resentment, alienation and anger can occur. If the sibling(s) can be included at initial meetings and discussions (on occasion, it may not be 'natural' for a family to include everyone) a lot of this conflict and subsequent trouble can be avoided, making the whole process less stressful for family and carers alike.

Obviously nurses can play a huge part in educating patients regarding their treatment details — where it's going, what is being done day-to-day and what reactions they can expect. A number of members made mention of the difference in information levels at inpatient and outpatient levels. It seems that there is a greater investment in the communication of procedure at outpatient level than at ward level. Perhaps this has its foundation in staffing ratios, time, individuals or repetition of procedures, but members who noticed certainly appreciated and welcomed the increased understanding of, and involvement in, their treatment while an outpatient.

The bottom line is that, as far as CanTeen Members are concerned, they can never know enough about what they or their sibling are going through. With knowledge they are empowered in the treatment process. It is very important for adolescents to have as much understanding and control over their environment as possible. Therefore it is important that every reasonable effort is made to involve them in their treatment. Once again nurses are the people in the best position to ensure that the communication and care that, hopefully, the doctors and specialists have started is supported and continued.

## CARE WHILE AN OUTPATIENT

All the members were overwhelmingly in favour of outpatient treatment and the benefits that this included —being able go home to sleep and interact, and having minimal disruption to everyday life. The controlling and clinical aspects of hospital life are seen as being as uncomfortable as the treatment itself.

One of the few negatives was a mention of some bias towards younger patients. The degree of care for patients under 12 is decidedly more than for those over 12. Several members felt that they were not being acknowledged where they otherwise might have been, and that this was based on their age. Once again it's difficult to differentiate between an adolescent's nose out of joint and a genuine bias, though this comment appeared in more than one state.

Overall being treated as an outpatient was by far the preferred treatment, probably because of the limited time for patients to reflect on what was going on. It was also recognised that nurses have to deal with a high turnover of patients and families, and need to be continually 'up' for this turnover.

## MULTICULTURAL PROVISION OF CARE

None of the respondents who were from another culture was given any literature in a language other than English that may have helped parents to better understand the patient's condition or treatment. It is understood that this is not the responsibility of the nursing staff but this sort of literature is bound to be needed and it would be interesting to look into where it may be obtained. None of the members perceived the lack of such literature as a problem, they merely commented that it was not provided.

# COMPLEMENTARY THERAPIES

It is pleasing to see nursing staff acknowledging complementary therapies (massage, aromatherapy, meditation etc.) although they do not appear to be actively promoted. No-one reported any denial of these activities; some simply did not receive them, while others were lucky enough to have them provided throughout their treatment. Most therapies are designed to relax the patient and to make the traumas of treatment and the stay in hospital easier to bear. It is pleasing that nursing staff are so open to minor detours outside the medical model.

In most, if not all, states CanTeen is able to provide most of the accepted complementary therapies and hospitals seeking such therapies could call their state's CanTeen office.

# EXTRA AND SUNDRY COMMENTS

There were a number of things that members commented on that we know are above and beyond the call of duty of oncology staff. The first of these was having nurses go out to schools to speak to classes and year levels about cancer and its treatment. In all cases this was seen to make a huge difference in the patient's ability to cope with school, in being accepted, and in no longer being seen as a *'freak'*. It is difficult enough educating those close to you let alone those people whom you may have little or nothing to do with. The issues of changes in appearance and people's general lack of understanding of cancer make it very uncomfortable for young people to involve themselves in any social setting, let alone the charged environment of school. This makes the hospitals' efforts at general education so much more important and valuable. These efforts are certainly valued by the patients and siblings in CanTeen.

A number of our female members commented on the value of courses and programs to boost low self-esteem while on treatment. Because of the radical changes to their appearance they commented that having access to make-overs and the like alleviates some of the negative self-image that accumulates during treatment. Obviously neither hospitals nor nurses can be held responsible for providing these, but if CanTeen or a similar support agency were approached, something could be arranged.

# SUMMARY

A lot of what has been described in this paper relates to different ways and means of helping young cancer patients feel better about themselves and what they are going through. There are also a number of things that, from an administrative angle, cannot be provided or changed by hospitals. These are, perhaps, areas where nursing staff might look to CanTeen for assistance. We are, after all, working together to provide 'total care' for young oncology patients and siblings who pass through Australia's hospitals.

However, there are a number of areas where, through acknowledgment and effort, improvement could be made. It is possible to increase the standard of overall care and to decrease the psychological discomfort of young people who are being treated for cancer. The people who see the daily interactions of the family, hear the problems and woes of the patients, notice dysfunctional families and recognise different pressures on individual patients are, of course, the nurses. If changes are to be made and things are to be acted on then it is often up to the nurses to initiate those changes.

This survey process that led to the publication of this paper was productive for both the patients and CanTeen as an organisation and we must congratulate oncology nurses for doing a very difficult and demanding job with incredible dedication and devotion.

# Index

## A

adaptation, 58, 62, 191
alternative therapies, 230
assessment, 5, 6, 11,16, 23, 33, 62, 78, 81,
   82, 96, 98, 99, 100, 109, 111, 112, 113,
   115, 119, 120, 121, 168, 194, 196, 201,
   224
attitude, 9, 55, 100, 112, 132, 165, 190,
   202, 224
autonomy, 98, 140, 144, 145, 193, 195, 206

## B

being, 4, 5, 6, 7, 9, 13, 22, 24, 27, 29, 32,
   34, 40, 44, 46, 52, 53, 54, 56, 59, 65, 66,
   75, 77, 78, 82, 89, 111, 113, 122, 124,
   125, 126, 127, 128, 129, 130, 131, 132,
   134, 140, 141, 143, 145, 149, 151, 152,
   155, 156, 157, 158, 164, 165, 168, 172,
   176, 178, 181, 182, 184, 190, 192, 193,
   195, 200, 203, 204, 205, 211, 214, 215,
   216, 221, 222, 224, 229, 233, 236, 237,
   238, 239, 240
breast cancer, 7, 36, 54, 58, 66, 72, 74, 79,
   80, 81, 84, 85, 86, 87, 89, 156, 176, 211,
   217, 218, 219, 220, 221, 222, 223, 224,
   225, 226, 227

## C

cancer pain, 88, 89, 90, 91, 92, 93, 94, 95,
   99, 100, 102, 103, 105, 106, 152, 158,
   186
caring, 3, 9, 28, 33, 46, 47, 58, 66, 80, 90,
   106, 112, 120, 123, 124, 125, 126, 127,
   128, 129, 130, 131, 132, 133, 134, 135,
   149, 150, 155, 156, 158, 160, 168, 175,
   176, 177, 179, 180, 184, 185, 188, 192,
   216
chronic pain, 91, 93, 96, 100, 105, 106
client, 3, 4, 5, 6, 7, 8, 9, 10, 17, 20, 22, 39,
   40, 43, 44, 45, 46, 83, 113, 174, 175,
   176, 178, 179, 180, 181, 182, 183, 184,
   185

clinical judgement, 110, 111, 119, 120
comfort, 9, 15, 28, 29, 30, 41, 44, 67, 73,
   81, 92, 94, 101, 104, 127, 128, 156, 157,
   163, 164, 166, 168, 176, 179, 180, 182,
   192, 202, 236
communication, 4, 6, 9, 10, 14, 15, 19, 27,
   30, 36, 37, 39, 40, 43, 45, 47, 65, 115,
   139, 140, 143, 157, 178, 179, 181, 182,
   190, 192, 193, 194, 195, 196, 225, 227,
   235, 238
complex physical therapy, 216
compliance, 82, 102, 104, 106, 207
concern, 7, 17, 18, 19, 23, 45, 59, 77, 80,
   83, 126, 127, 132, 156, 169, 170, 179,
   182, 201, 214, 222
coping, 16, 30, 31, 33, 42, 53, 56, 57, 58,
   59, 60, 62, 99, 110, 115, 120, 133, 149,
   151, 155, 159, 179, 183, 189, 191, 232,
   233, 236
counselling, 14, 33, 35, 36, 78, 80, 81, 82,
   83, 84, 106, 145, 206

## D

death, 13, 14, 16, 29, 33, 34, 35, 36, 40,
   45, 51, 54, 55, 57, 61,64, 65, 90, 93, 94,
   130, 134, 149, 150, 153, 154, 155, 157,
   159, 164, 167, 172, 174, 175, 176, 178,
   179, 180, 182, 183, 184, 185, 190, 191,
   218, 221, 222, 225, 229
debrief, 35, 177, 178, 179
discharge planning, 6, 100, 113

## E

education, 2, 3, 4, 7, 8, 9, 10, 13, 14, 15,
   17, 18, 19, 20, 21, 22, 23, 24, 25, 26,
   30, 38, 40, 50, 73, 78, 81, 88, 90, 100,
   105, 106, 108, 111, 113, 114, 137, 139,
   143, 146, 159, 174, 178, 183, 185, 186,
   188, 195, 198, 201, 202, 203, 225,
   229, 239
embarrassment, 9, 44, 67, 81, 213, 215
empowerment, 5, 58, 130, 195, 228, 229

encouragement, 59, 164, 184, 201, 205
ethical behaviours, 137, 138
ethical decision-making, 139, 141, 147
ethical dilemma, 138, 139, 141, 147
ethical problem, 138, 139, 140, 141
ethical skills, 141
ethics rounds, 146
evaluation, 3, 106, 111, 224, 226, 228,
    230, 234

**F**

faith, 127, 150, 154, 155, 156, 157
family, 4, 7, 9, 13, 16, 21, 27, 28, 29, 30,
    34, 35, 36, 45, 46, 57, 60, 65, 66, 77, 78,
    80, 90, 112, 113, 114, 118, 124, 125,
    126, 127, 129, 130, 131, 132, 139, 142,
    143, 144, 145, 146, 151, 152, 153, 154,
    155, 164, 165, 167, 168, 172, 179, 189,
    191, 192, 194, 203, 206, 214, 221, 222,
    234, 236, 237, 240
family planning, 80
fears, 33, 45, 49, 114, 170, 190, 215, 216,
    218, 220, 221, 222, 223, 225
feelings, 28, 33, 34, 35, 42, 45, 54, 58, 59,
    66, 67, 78, 96, 114, 125, 129, 130, 132,
    141, 150, 152, 154, 156, 176, 189, 191,
    195, 218, 219, 222, 225
fertility, 31, 69, 74, 75, 79, 82, 83, 85
focus of care, 166, 168
fostering hope, 154
future, 10, 15, 19, 20, 22, 24, 30, 39, 40,
    45, 52, 53, 55, 57, 61, 74, 77, 78, 79, 80,
    82, 112, 119, 122, 132, 134, 136, 145,
    146, 147, 153, 154, 198, 199, 200, 201,
    202, 205, 207, 215

**G**

Gonadal dysfunction, 69, 71, 75, 76
grief, 16, 28, 30, 35, 164, 175, 176, 177,
    178, 179, 180, 182, 184, 189

**H**

health, 3, 5, 10, 13, 15, 17, 18, 19, 23, 26,
    27, 28, 30, 31, 34, 35, 39, 40, 46, 51, 54,
    56, 58, 60, 62, 66, 67, 72, 73, 77, 80, 81,
    82, 84, 92, 93, 110, 112, 113, 114, 121,
    123, 127, 130, 131, 137, 138, 139, 140,
    141, 142, 143, 144, 145, 151, 152, 159,
    164, 165, 166, 168, 169, 170, 171, 172,
    174, 176, 177, 180, 183, 188, 189, 190,
    191, 192, 193, 194, 195, 196, 198, 199,
    200, 201, 202, 203, 204, 205, 207, 210,
    211, 215, 216, 219, 221, 224, 225, 229,
    230, 233
health care needs, 211, 216
Heidegger, 126, 130, 132, 134
holistic care, 149
hope, 3, 9, 10, 29, 40, 45, 51, 52, 53, 54,
    55, 56, 57, 58, 59, 60, 61, 62, 63, 78,
    127, 129, 150, 152, 153, 154, 158, 165,
    168, 170, 172, 190
hopefulness, 37, 54, 60, 61, 62
hopelessness, 54, 59, 61, 153, 191
hospice, 14, 34, 50, 56, 159, 163, 164,
    165, 169

**I**

infection, 16, 82, 117, 118, 211, 213
information, 3, 4, 5, 6, 8, 10, 15, 19, 20,
    26, 27, 28, 29, 30, 31, 32, 34, 35, 36,
    37, 41, 42, 43, 44, 54, 58, 59, 69, 73,
    74, 80, 83, 84, 92, 93, 94, 98, 100,
    109, 110, 111, 112, 114, 115, 119, 125,
    139, 142, 143, 144, 145, 146, 154, 182,
    183, 189, 193, 194, 195, 200, 201, 204,
    205, 212, 216, 225, 231, 232, 234, 235,
    237, 238
Initial assessment, 114

**K**

knowing the patient, 110, 111, 112, 117,
    119, 121
knowledge, 3, 4, 5, 6, 8, 9, 14, 15, 17, 19,
    22, 23, 41, 43, 56, 57, 74, 81, 82, 89, 93,
    100, 102, 110, 111, 112, 113, 115, 119,
    120, 140, 146, 156, 157, 164, 172, 179,
    189, 201, 206, 225, 227, 238

**L**

learning, 3, 5, 6, 7, 9, 14, 18, 19, 20, 22,
    23, 24, 113, 132, 189, 202, 206
lifestyle, 16, 32, 33, 72, 77, 84, 91, 188,
    189, 216, 228, 229, 233
lived experience, 86, 126, 133, 134

loneliness, 222, 228
lymphoedema, 210, 211, 212, 213, 214,
   215, 216, 217

**M**

mammography, 207, 218, 220, 226
mastectomy, 215, 218, 220, 221, 224, 226
meaning, 29, 52, 58, 62, 96, 110, 123, 124,
   126, 132, 133, 149, 150, 151, 152, 153,
   155, 156, 157, 158, 159, 163, 188, 191,
   192
menopause, 71, 72, 73, 75, 78, 85,
   86, 87
myelosuppression, 115, 116

**N**

non-maleficence, 138, 143, 144
nutrition, 2, 31, 38, 98, 115, 118

**O**

oncology nurse, 5, 9, 10, 21, 24, 59, 82,
   84, 109, 112, 116, 125, 126, 127, 128,
   129, 130, 132, 133, 149, 158, 174,
   176, 177, 178, 179, 180, 202, 205,
   225, 240
ovum, 78

**P**

pain, 33, 89, 90, 91, 94, 95, 102, 105, 106,
   214, 223
pain assessment, 56, 96, 98
pain control, 88, 93, 96, 98, 100, 101, 105,
   166, 186
palliative care, 12, 16, 19, 20, 33, 34,
   50, 57, 99, 106, 148, 162, 163, 164,
   165, 166, 167, 168, 169, 170, 171,
   172
patient rights, 140, 144
personal rewards, 131, 132, 153
phenomenology, 121, 126, 133
physical needs, 129
positive outcomes, 228
postgraduate, 13, 17, 18, 20, 137, 148
pregnancy, 79, 80, 81, 84
programs, 5, 9, 10, 14, 18, 21, 24, 28,
   34, 88, 186, 195, 200, 212, 218, 225,
   239

**Q**

quality of life, 31, 33, 40, 62, 66, 81, 85,
   96, 99, 102, 138, 144, 152, 155, 159,
   166, 172, 214, 216, 229

**R**

rapport, 4, 30, 32, 46
recurrence, 32, 33, 74, 80, 81, 118, 215,
   228, 229, 232
relaxation, 58, 73, 101, 180, 228, 229, 230,
   231, 232, 233

**S**

'screaming room', 46
self-concept, 4, 118
self-esteem, 4, 66, 67, 132, 239
sexual health, 65, 67, 74, 76, 78, 82, 83,
   84
sexuality, 16, 31, 65, 66, 67, 71, 72, 74,
   76, 77, 81, 82, 83, 86, 87
significant other, 46, 174, 175, 176, 177,
   179, 180, 181, 182, 183, 184, 185
skin, 67, 72, 75, 78, 92, 101, 115, 116, 117,
   118, 207, 211, 219
sperm, 69, 78, 79, 82
spiritual dimension, 149, 150, 151, 157,
   158, 159
spiritual needs, 149, 151, 155, 156,
   158, 159
spirituality, 33, 62, 148, 149, 150, 151, 155,
   156, 157, 158, 159
stress, 10, 28, 35, 39, 72, 73, 82, 113, 129,
   141, 155, 170, 177, 180, 225, 228, 229,
   230, 231, 232, 233
suffering, 91
support, 5, 6, 9, 10, 13, 19, 20, 23,
   24, 26, 28, 29, 30, 31, 32, 33, 34,
   35, 36, 37, 40, 44, 45, 46, 53, 54,
   58, 59, 60, 73, 74, 92, 100, 112,
   113, 118, 124, 125, 127, 129,
   140, 145, 151, 154, 155, 156,
   158, 159, 163, 164, 170, 172,
   175, 176, 177, 178, 179, 180,
   181, 182, 183, 184, 185, 203,
   224, 225, 228, 229, 230, 231, 232,
   233, 239
symptom management, 16

## T

teaching, 4, 5, 6, 9, 10, 13, 15,20, 23, 50,
    88, 100, 124, 174, 186, 207, 214, 234
terminal illness, 52, 60, 163, 166
themes, 126, 127, 236
traditions, 124, 166, 172, 190

## U

undergraduate, 15, 17, 20, 137